Passing the UK Clinical Aptitude Test and BMAT

Third edition

Passing the UK Clinical Aptitude Test and BMAT

Felicity Taylor, Rosalie Hutton and Glenn Hutton

Third edition

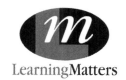

LearningMatters

Published by Learning Matters
33 Southernhay East
Exeter EX1 1NX
Tel: 01392 215560
info@learningmatters.co.uk
www.learningmatters.co.uk

First published in 2006
Reprinted in 2006 (twice)
Second edition published in 2007
Reprinted in 2007 (three times)
Third edition published in 2008

British Cataloguing-in-Publication Data

A catalogue record for this book is available from the British Library.

ISBN 978 1 84445 178 4

Typeset by Pantek Arts Ltd, Maidstone, Kent

Printed by Bell & Bain Ltd, Glasgow

Contents

10. The Abstract Reasoning subtest

11. The Decision Analysis subtest

12. The Non-Cognitive Analysis subtest

Part III: Preparing for the BioMedical Admissions Test (BMAT)

Felicity Taylor

13. BMAT Section 1: Aptitude and Skills

Acknowledgements

The publisher and authors would like to thank the following for permission to reproduce extracts:

The British Psychological Society – Extract from Patrick Packwood, 'Enabling dyslexics to cope in employment' (2006) *Selection & Development Review* 22(1).

Guardian Newspapers Limited – Extract from Randeep Ramesh, 'Drug firms seek to stop generic HIV treatment', 11 May 2006.

Oxford University Press – Extract from Fraser Sampson, Blackstone's Police Manual, Volume 4, *General Police Duties* (2005).

The Times – Extract from Tony Halpin, 'Degrees in two years to ease student debt burden', 18 April 2006.

Every effort has been made to contact copyright holders for their permission to reproduce extracts contained in this book. Apologies are offered for any errors or omissions, which will be rectified in future editions.

FT: To my parents and Damian

RH and GH: To the memory of Martin Orme

Part I
Introduction

Chapter 1
The tests

Over the past few years, there has been a shift towards a more detailed assessment of students applying to university, in order to best discover their suitability for studying at undergraduate level. Nowhere has this extra burden of assessment been felt more keenly than in applying to read medicine, dentistry and veterinary science/medicine: due to the huge numbers of high-quality applicants competing for each available place, with often nothing to choose between candidates in terms of exam results, the schools have turned towards alternative methods of assessing candidates' aptitudes. The first test to come into existence was the BioMedical Admissions Test (BMAT), which combines aptitude tests with an assessment of scientific knowledge and reasoning skills. At the six medical and veterinary schools that currently use the BMAT, it has proved very successful in providing a more in-depth description of candidates' strengths and weaknesses, allowing admissions officers to use this information as part of their selection process.

The second (and latest) test that has been developed is the UK Clinical Aptitude Test (UKCAT). The UKCAT aims to test verbal reasoning, quantitative reasoning, abstract reasoning and decision analysis rather than scientific knowledge. Unlike its cousin the BMAT, the UKCAT has been taken up by the majority of UK medical schools and some dentistry schools, so it is likely that, if you are intending to apply to university to read medicine or dentistry, you will have to sit the UKCAT. This is the third year of the UKCAT and, for most candidates, it remains somewhat of a mystery and is creating a large amount of anxiety. Some candidates will have to sit both the BMAT and UKCAT and may feel unsure how they will manage to prepare for both tests while still keeping up with their normal studies.

This book has been designed to assist you prepare for both the BMAT and UKCAT exams by helping you to familiarise yourself with the types of questions used, and how to solve them. The developers of both the BMAT and UKCAT advise that their tests cannot be revised for, but it is certain that they can definitely be prepared for: a familiarity with what you will meet in the test and a knowledge of what is required of you, combined with confidence in answering the questions, will enable you to fulfil your full potential and will remove a lot of the unnecessary anxiety and stress these tests generate.

The first part of this book contains advice and practical support on applying to medical school, taking you through the application process step by step, including details on how to write your personal statement, how to arrange work experience and how to succeed in interviews.

In Part II of this book you will find detailed instructions on how to prepare for the UKCAT exam, including analysis of the types of questions you will encounter, practice tests and worked examples so that you can understand where mistakes are made and how to avoid them yourself.

Finally, Part III tackles the BMAT, providing examples and exam-style tests so that you can familiarise yourself with the standard required and build your confidence prior to the test. In this part there is also a detailed discussion regarding the essay section, with tips on how to research, plan and write the perfect essay.

At the beginning of many chapters there are a number of learning objectives, allowing you to monitor your progress and tackle your preparation in bite-size chunks.

While this book cannot promise you a guaranteed pass on the UKCAT and BMAT, if you follow the advice it offers and practise the questions it contains, we can promise that you will be much better prepared for the tests – which will permit you to achieve your best possible result.

Good luck with the tests and your future career!

Chapter 2
So just why do you want to be a doctor?

This chapter will help you to:

- consider why you want to study at medical school
- consider why you want a career as a doctor.

Congratulations – you've decided to choose a career in medicine. 'So, just why do you want to be a doctor?' How many times have you heard that one already? Whether you've 'just known' since you were knee high to a grasshopper or this has been a recent development, it's the one question that you can guarantee you'll be asked by friends, family, teachers. No other choice for a degree course seems to trigger so much curiosity. Perhaps this is a hangover from the days when doctors were omnipotent and commanding, or perhaps due to a general fascination as to why anyone might want to cut up dead people as part of his or her degree course. Whatever the reason, this constant questioning begins to be a bit wearing after a while, especially if, just like I did, you feel something of a fake because you have no real answer to this apparently vital question.

I did, however, have lots of answers which sounded good, or ones that I thought I was supposed to say. To give you just a few, I wanted 'to help people', 'to apply my scientific knowledge to disease' and to 'serve the community'. Now, I'm not ridiculing these ideals, but if you really went into your medical degree with these in mind then you wouldn't last too long. Surely you would be helping people far more if you went and dug some water mains in Africa rather than spending your time languishing in the library of some veritable medical institution? I would instead suggest that the question 'why do you want to be a doctor?' is unfair, because it assumes personal knowledge of a career that you cannot possibly have yet. For example, no one has ever asked the question of a prospective accountant 'why do you want to be an accountant' and received the answer 'because I like sitting in an office and chasing up tax accounts'.

People choose a career because they are interested in the subject on which it is based. You could study law at university and end up in any manner of jobs; you may only choose to become a solicitor or barrister because what you have studied during your degree interested you enough to spend the rest of your life doing it. The same goes for medicine, but the difference is that, because it costs so much and takes so long to train a doctor, they are interviewing you for your job on your entry to university, rather than at the end.

This is perhaps why the choice seems so important: unlike a degree in biology, you are saying to yourself and the world: 'This is what I am going to be doing for the rest of my life.' At such a tender age I found it impossible to imagine a career at 30 and beyond, so at this stage it is more practical for you to focus on why you want to go to medical school and study medicine, and then consider whether you actually fancy being a doctor at the end of it all.

So why do you want to go to medical school?

At medical school you will study pretty much everything and anything to do with the human body and the human mind. So you'd better like your human biology module at A-level otherwise you'll be in for a rough ride. Just some of the basic science subjects you will come across during your degree include physiology, anatomy, biochemistry, pharmacology, sociology, psychology, genetics, neuroscience, pathology, histology and immunology, and that's even before you get to the clinical specialties like cardiology, gynaecology, etc. That's a lot of learning.

If the thought of spending days absorbed in books before you even get near a living person sounds quite appealing, and you're quite prepared to spend the next 15 years of your life sitting exams, then medicine is clearly the choice for you. For the rest of us, during moments of self-doubt, we can take a step back and consider how truly wonderful it would be to understand how our own bodies work; to understand everything from how our skin protects us from the elements to how our cells turn our Weetabix into a sprint for the bus. We can't escape from ourselves, and you will find that your own body acts as a constant reminder of how little you know and how much you have yet to discover. Which is actually pretty exciting, especially for intelligent, knowledge-seeking people like yourselves.

However, you will be pleased to hear that there is plenty to do at medical school besides study. You may think that your extracurricular activities will stop as soon as you get your place, but, actually, with the new modernising medical careers programme for junior doctors now up and running, it is more important than ever that you get involved in activities and organisations in order to continue your development as a well rounded individual.

At medical school you will probably find the most diverse range of people in any degree course in the country, all with a single ambition. So, depending on the size of the medical school, you will instantly have up to 450 new best friends! After all the struggle to get to medical school you will find it is a surprisingly supportive and uncompetitive place, and I promise that you will love it. There will certainly be times when you think you can't continue, but they soon pass and they actually serve to make you even more determined.

Why do you think you want a job as a doctor?

Some of you may have decided long ago that medicine was for you and, if so, you deserve congratulations for picking such a great career so early on. Others of you may have personal experience of family members working in medicine. If either of these apply, you'll have realised by now that a career in medicine has a few downsides: the constant exams, the endless lists of knowledge, the late nights, the early mornings, the slow career progression, the constant moving around, the abusive patients… I could go on.

So what makes the very brightest of us want to sacrifice a large proportion of our best years to a job like this? If you think about it, there are a lot of reasons. First, can you think of any other job where you get up each day not having a clue about what you will see, whom you will meet and who or what will come flying at you through the door?

Secondly, you will never get bored because medicine has an incredibly varying routine, limited only by the variety of people in the world. Plus, as you'll never know everything, you can't stagnate: medicine is constantly changing and adapting as new knowledge is added. Thirdly, to the nitty gritty: money. There seems to be some unwritten rule that 'thou shalt not discuss money or working conditions when thou art a prospective medical student'. I don't know why this is. Perhaps it doesn't fit with the self-sacrificing image we think we have to portray in order to get into medical school, but all the same the pay isn't bad.

No one who becomes a doctor is going to get rich quick, but you're not going to be out on the streets either. At present, a newly qualified junior doctor in a 'high intensity post' (that means working your fingers to the bone and doing lots of extra hours) can expect to take home about £30,000. You also have very little potential to be unemployed unless you want to be, and you'll also get an excellent pension. Luckily, the NHS has also got its act together as regards flexible training (that's part-time work in non-NHS speak), so your career won't suffer if you want to have a family (you might not be thinking about that one at the moment, but you'll be glad of it in later years!).

If you weren't convinced before, I'm sure you are now. All that remains for you to do is to get that coveted place at medical school. You are probably aware that a few hurdles lie in your way between now and then, namely, excellent A-level grades, a fantastic personal statement, a resounding score on the BMAT or UKCAT exam and, finally, a jaw-dropping performance at interview. And there's the competition – have a look at Table 1 for the 2006 year of entry to UK medical schools to see what you're up against.

Table 1 Entry to UK medical schools (2006)

	All applications	All acceptances	Clearing acceptances	Acceptances (per cent)
Men	8,379	3,309	168	41.5
Women	10,570	4,702	212	46.5
Total	18,949	8,011	380	44.2

A glance at these figures shows that the competition is pretty fierce, but it shouldn't put you off. You have as much chance as anyone else and, if you follow the advice and preparation outlined in this book, together with some hard work practising for either the BMAT and/or the UKCAT, you can be fairly confident that you will be as good as they get, if not better.

The next chapter outlines the stages in your application to read medicine in the UK, and the following chapters contain practical advice and tips for each of the stages you will go through. If at any time you feel that this is all a lot of extra work and a bit too stressful in comparison with what your friends are having to go through for their respective degree courses, I would advise returning to this section to remind yourself just why you want to study medicine; suddenly everything will seem much more in proportion.

Chapter 3
Your application to read medicine: step by step

This chapter will help you to:

- plan your application from start to finish
- organise your time
- keep your application on track.

The fact you're reading this is perhaps proof that the last chapter did not put you off a career in medicine! As a reward for your commitment, this chapter will help to steer you through all the different parts of your application to medical school, providing you with key dates and deadlines and a suggested timescale for events to help you to keep stress levels down and success levels high. You will find detailed information on each of these stages in the chapters that follow, but you can refer back to this chapter at any time to see how it all slots together.

Those of you who are that way inclined can even tick each stage off as you go along – it may seem a small reward for all the work you are putting in, but keep concentrating on your end goal: to become a doctor. Make sure you involve everyone you can to help with your application: teachers have a wealth of experience and will be delighted to help an enthusiastic student, and your family will provide much needed emotional and moral support during times of stress. Most of all, remember that, while getting into medical school is important, it isn't as important as your health and happiness, so make time for relaxation, friends and the things you enjoy.

Key dates for your diary 2008–2009

2008

May
1   UKCAT online registration opens for all applicants entering medical school in 2009, or deferred entry for 2010
Register online at www.ukcat.ac.uk

July
7   UKCAT exam opens at test centres
Medical school open days
Register to sit the BMAT – details online at www.bmat.org.uk

August
16   Publication of A1 results

September
1   UCAS application procedure opens
26   UKCAT registration closes
30   Closing date for BMAT exam applications

October
10   Closing date for UKCAT test sittings
15   Late-entry closing date for BMAT (fee payable)
15   Deadline for UCAS applications for Oxford and Cambridge, and medicine, dentistry and veterinary science or veterinary medicine

November
5   BMAT exam
30   BMAT results published

December
Cambridge University interviews
Oxford University interviews
Oxford University offers/rejections

2009

January
Cambridge University offers/rejections
Cambridge University 'pool'
11   Closing date for BMAT results

February
Medical school interviews and offers/rejections

March
31   Deadline for declining or accepting all your offers

May–June
A-level exams

August
Publication of A2 results; Clearing opens
Offers confirmed by universities

September–October
Start medical school!

Preparation timeline

May–August
Practise UKCAT questions before test
Work on personal statement – first and second drafts
Arrange work experience/voluntary work
Choose an area of interest to read around
Attend university open days
Research medical schools

September
Final decision on medical schools and non-medical degree choices
Final draft of personal statement for checking by your teacher
Complete UCAS form and hand in

October–November
Start preparation for BMAT exam
Continue work on area of interest

Keep up to date with topical medical news

December–February
Prepare for upcoming interviews
Monitor offers/rejections via UCAS website

March onwards
Continue working for A-level exams
Make decisions regarding acceptances/next steps after rejection

Chapter 4
Preparing to apply to medical school

This chapter will help you to:

- decide if medicine is the right course for you
- choose the right medical school and course
- collect evidence for your UCAS personal statement.

While it is never too late to decide to study medicine at university, your application will certainly benefit from an early start. With over 19,000 students competing for a mere 8,000 places at medical school last year, you can see the competition is fierce. These days, applying to study medicine is a lot tougher than it was even just a few years ago: not only do you have to have the top grades at GCSE and A-level, but you must also achieve a good mark on the UKCAT and/or the BMAT exam. In addition, you must produce a well-rounded personal statement that shows evidence of work experience, a variety of extracurricular activities and a keen interest in scientific matters.

It is, then, perhaps not so surprising that students who have decided early on that they want to apply to medical school always ask me what things they can do to improve their chances. Whether you have yet to sit your GCSE exams or have just started your A-level courses, it's not too early to start preparing your application (as long as you don't neglect your other studies to do it). You will find that a little time invested now will make your life so much easier when the time comes around to apply.

This chapter offers practical tips and advice for preparing all aspects of your application to medical school, along with resources and suggested timeframes to ensure you get the very best result from your application. For those of you with a little less time on your hands, all these tips can be adapted to the time you have available; you might just have to work that bit harder!

Important note: It is also vital to remember that medical schools are not looking for a certain 'type' of person; nor are they looking to produce an army of doctor clones! They want to train students who are intelligent, enthusiastic, committed and driven. So don't feel that you ever have to do something that you don't want to because it's 'needed' for medical school – all these suggestions are just ways of demonstrating to the admissions officers what an ideal candidate for medical school you really are!

Deciding if medicine really is for you

All medical schools want to be sure that they won't be spending five years and a huge amount of government money training you, only for you to leave after a few years, having decided medicine really isn't your cup of tea after all. Similarly, you are going to have to make a choice relatively early on in your life about how you want to spend the rest of it – this isn't something to be taken lightly! Luckily, there are lots of things you can do to research careers in medicine, and you may be surprised to find out about the variety of other careers in the NHS and non-medical professions: there are, after all, lots of other jobs which involve science and healthcare, such as pharmacy, occupational therapy, physiotherapy. It is worth considering whether these alternative careers would suit you better. Even if this research only serves to make you more determined to become a doctor, then they're worth a look, especially as you will have to choose two non-medical school choices on your UCAS application form as 'insurance'.

Exam results

Unfortunately, there's no getting away from it: to study medicine you have to be smart, and you have to prove it by achieving good grades. Before you decide whether you want to be a doctor, it's best to be realistic and look at your chances based on your GCSE grades and your predicted or actual A1 module results. To give you some idea of what you need to achieve, have a look at the requirements below of a typical medical school. You need these results as an absolute minimum; many students will have grades in excess of this. (If you don't quite measure up, either in grades or subjects, don't give up straightaway: have a look at the section on page 16 on access schemes and do some research to see if you could get on a foundation or entry programme to medicine.)

Minimum requirements
GCSEs
■ At least six grade As to include chemistry, biology and physics (or Science Dual Award).
■ Grade A at AS-level physics can compensate for a B at GCSE level.
■ Minimum of grade B in maths and English language.

AS and A2
Biology and chemistry passed at grade A and a third subject (excluding general studies) passed at grade B.

NB: Scottish Highers, International Baccalaureate and the Irish Leaving Certificate are all valid qualifications. Check with your intended medical school for precise requirements.

Finding out about life as a doctor

There is obviously no point in going to medical school if you don't think you would like life as a doctor. It can be quite hard to get an idea of what the daily grind and boring details (such as pay, hours, work schedule) will be like before you actually start the job. There are lots of resources on the NHS careers website (see the useful contacts section below), including job descriptions for doctors and other healthcare professionals, advice on what medical schools are looking for in prospective students, outlines of possible career pathways, and details of pay and working conditions. You can also order a free NHS careers publication, *Becoming a Doctor in the NHS*, online. This is well worth a look before you jump headfirst into the application process.

Also worth a look is the website of the British Medical Association (BMA). Although primarily for medical students and doctors, there are lots of useful links and descriptions of characteristics required to succeed in medicine (especially useful for writing your personal statement).

Medicine simulation courses

A number of companies offer courses, often over two or more days, where you can experience what it would be like to be a doctor (see the useful contacts section below). These courses are a mixture of lectures and practical sessions led by doctors and academics, and they offer you the chance to meet other potential medical students and to get a flavour of what it is like to wear surgical scrubs, hang a stethoscope around your neck and talk to patients. For a lot of students who are considering medicine, this is a fun way to spend a couple of days – it's a little like a school trip – and it confirms for most students that this is indeed what they want to do rather than being an off-putting experience. However, the courses tend to be during July and at the University of Nottingham, which may be difficult for some of you to attend.

I am always asked by students and their parents whether this type of course is worth the expense (courses tend to start at around £200 and can get increasingly pricey if you add in all the extras they offer). Personally, I never went on one of these courses, and this didn't do me any harm, but if you fancy going and you have the money to spare, then it's probably worth it for the experience. Just be aware that they tend to make a lot of fuss about it being a really great thing to put on your UCAS personal statement and that it will give you an edge in a competitive application process. As you will see later (see Chapter 6), it isn't what you have done, but what you have learnt from it.

Going on one of these courses is just another piece of evidence that you have considered medicine as a career, but admissions officers recognise the courses for what they are and won't give you any credit for attending one unless you can demonstrate what you have learnt from it. Similarly, don't feel that you will be penalised if you can't make it to one or can't afford to go; you absolutely, definitely, won't be.

University access schemes

Perhaps you're not sure if medicine is for you. You think you don't have the right grades, the right social background; you might even be wondering whether you can afford to go to medical school at all. For a long time, students with these sort of doubts were put off going to medical school but, over the last few years, many of the schools have been actively recruiting local students who are from non-traditional backgrounds or who have slightly lower grades to attend access, information or workshop events aimed at recruiting the very best students with the greatest potential. Eventually, if these students decide to apply to medical school, there are a variety of entry programmes, ranging from qualifying years to catch-up courses, to enable them to study.

Recruitment for these schemes tends to be at local school level, with activities starting from pre-GCSE onwards, so you should check with your local medical school or look at their website if you think this type of activity might help you. For example, King's College London offer an extended medical degree for students living in certain London boroughs who would not normally qualify for the standard medical degree; look at their website for more details (see the useful contacts section below).

Useful contacts
Finding out about life as a doctor
- www.nhscareers.nhs.uk – NHS careers website.
- www.bma.org.uk – website of the British Medical Association. Contains lots of information about medical schools and future training pathways.

Medicine simulation courses
- www.medlink-uk.com/ – more information about the Medsim and Medlink courses; aimed at students who have decided on a career as a doctor.
- http://www.workshop-uk.com/medisix.php – more information on the Medisix courses, which are for those of you who are interested in a career in medicine, dentistry, radiography or research.
- www.rsm.ac.uk – the Royal Society of Medicine sometimes has lectures and activity days aimed at prospective medical students. Check the website diary regularly for upcoming events or become a member to receive more information.

University access schemes

http://www.kcl.ac.uk/ugpo8/programme687 – access website for the King's College London medical school. Also contains details about the extended medical degree programme for students who do not have classical A-level entry grades and who live in one of the London borough catchment areas.

Deciding where you want to go

Medical schools

There are over 30 medical schools in the UK, and you are able to choose up to four to apply to via your UCAS form, plus two non-medical degree courses. If you start early with considering your university choices, you can really get a feel for which ones you would like to apply for. At an early stage it's best to visit each of the medical school websites; these vary in quality and content but generally have lots of information on required grades, course structures, life as a student, etc. (For ease of reference, I have included a list of all of the medical school websites in the useful contacts section below.)

After you have decided which medical schools take your fancy, you'll probably want to visit them to get a real feel for the place. The easiest way to do this is to attend one of their open days, which are generally held over the summer holidays. You can often attend lectures, speak to students and have tours of the accommodation blocks. It's really important that you choose your medical school based on the 'feel' of it and the course structure, rather than on rumours you have heard about it being 'hard' or 'easy' to get into. The best way to ignore these whisperings is to focus on which schools you want to apply to and then concentrate on making your application as polished as you can.

At this point you may feel that you'd be happy to get in just about anywhere, but five or six years is a long time to spend in a place that you find you can't stand! Also note the difference in course structure. For example, at Oxford and Cambridge you can transfer to another medical school (usually Oxbridge or London) after the first three years, and at St Andrews you can move to Manchester to complete your clinical degree period. Different courses have different advantages and disadvantages, and only you can decide which ones seem right for you.

Graduate entry and foundation courses

Medical schools are now being more flexible in their approach to medical school entry, allowing graduates from other degree disciplines and students who don't have the traditional or necessary qualifications to apply for places through graduate entry (typically four-year programmes) and foundation course schemes (typically an extra year on top of the standard course). The universities offering these options are listed below (see their websites for further details). Bear in mind that competition for entry to these programmes is even fiercer (if that's possible) than that of standard programmes. To succeed, you'll have to show an even greater level of commitment, desire and determination than the rest of us!

Foundation year entry courses
University of Bristol
University of Cardiff
University of Dundee
University of Edinburgh
King's College London (University of London)
University of Manchester
University of Sheffield
University of Southampton

Graduate entry courses
University of Birmingham
University of Bristol
University of Cambridge
Cardiff University
Imperial College, London
Keele University
King's College London (University of London)
University of Leicester
University of Liverpool
University of Newcastle upon Tyne
University of Nottingham
Oxford University
Queen Mary, University of London
St George's, University of London
Swansea University
University of Southampton
University of Warwick

Useful contacts
Medical schools
http://www.chms.ac.uk – the Council of Heads of Medical Schools website. Contains links to all the UK medical schools and also details of foundation and graduate entry courses.

University of Aberdeen (http://www.abdn.ac.uk/)
University of Birmingham (http://www.bham.ac.uk/)
Brighton and Sussex Medical School (http://www.bsms.ac.uk/)
University of Bristol (http://www.bris.ac.uk/)

University of Cambridge (http://www.cam.ac.uk/)
University of Dundee (http://www.dundee.ac.uk/)
University of East Anglia (http://www.med.uea.ac.uk/)
University of Edinburgh (http://www.ed.ac.uk/)
University of Glasgow (http://www.gla.ac.uk/)
Hull York Medical School (http://www.hyms.ac.uk/)
Imperial College London (University of London) (http://www.imperial.ac.uk/)
Keele University (http://www.keele.ac.uk/)
King's College London (University of London) (http://www.kcl.ac.uk/)
University of Leeds (http://www.leeds.ac.uk/)
University of Leicester (http://www.le.ac.uk)
University of Liverpool (http://www.liv.ac.uk/Medicine)
University of Manchester (http://www.manchester.ac.uk/)
University of Newcastle upon Tyne (http://www.ncl.ac.uk/)
University of Nottingham (http://www.nottingham.ac.uk/)
Oxford University (http://www.medsci.ox.ac.uk/)
Peninsula Medical School (http://www.pms.ac.uk/pms/)
Queen Mary, University of London (http://www.smd.qmul.ac.uk/)
Queen's University Belfast (http://www.qub.ac.uk/)
University of St Andrews (Medical Science BSc) (http://www.st-andrews.ac.uk/)
St George's, University of London (http://www.sgul.ac.uk/)
University of Sheffield (http://www.shef.ac.uk/)
University of Southampton (http://www.soton.ac.uk/)
University College London (University of London)
   (http://www.ucl.ac.uk/medicalschool/)
University of Wales (http://www.cardiff.ac.uk)
University of Wales, Swansea (http://www.swansea.ac.uk)
University of Warwick (graduate entry programme) (http://www2.warwick.ac.uk/)

Preparing to write your personal statement

When you read Chapter 6, you'll realise just how important your personal statement is for your application to medicine. There are very definite items that need to go on your personal statement, including evidence of academic commitment to medicine, work experience and extracurricular achievements. Obviously, life is going to be extremely difficult for you when you come to write your personal statement if you haven't actually done anything worth mentioning during your time at school or college.

If you are still a while off applying to university, then you have loads of time to get involved with lots of activities and to read around your subject. If your application deadline is fast approaching, then you need to be organised. Please note that it isn't about doing activities just so you have something to put on your form (although this is infinitely better than lying about non-existent voluntary work!) but, rather, a focused way of showing off your talents and suitability for medicine. However, as a general rule, I find that driven people like you tend to be pretty involved in school or college life, so you may only need a little extra help in one or two areas.

Work experience

First, you need to do some sort of work experience in order to demonstrate some knowledge and understanding of the profession you will be training to enter. This is easy if you know someone who works as a doctor but much harder for those of you who don't, especially if you're starting early and are relatively young to be rattling around in a doctor's surgery.

If you have a friend or relative who can help to arrange some work experience for you, think carefully about what you would like to do. Obviously, everyone wants to run down the corridor screaming 'get me the epinephrine' just like in *ER*, but it's not going to happen, and to be honest you'd be better off concentrating on talking to junior doctors, students, even your GP, and finding out what they think of the health service and medicine in general. Please, always remember that people's experiences in medicine vary wildly.

If you don't have a friendly doctor to hand, then your first port of call is your school careers adviser. Often, this person can arrange a placement for you with the minimum of fuss. If that does not work, then contact your local hospital and see if they can accommodate you for any work experience. Many hospital trusts offer programmes which involve either a day shadowing a doctor or as an observer in a specific department. Check the websites of your local NHS trust but note that it's best to inquire very early as these places get snapped up quickly.

Also bear in mind that a lot of schemes will only take students in their final year of A-levels and will sometimes keep you on a waiting list for months. Again, apply early as you wouldn't want to miss being able to write about your experience on your form.

Students often ask me whether they will be penalised if they haven't been able to organise any medical work experience, and the answer to that is a resounding 'No'. While it is preferable to try to get some experience, tutors realise the difficulty in arranging it and indeed expect that you will also demonstrate other ways of finding out about medicine, such as talking to doctors or researching career pathways on the Internet. In fact, some medical schools, such as the University of Leicester, actually state that medical work experience is not essential, while others state that, if you do say you've done some work experience, you will be asked about it at interview – so you better have something good to say about it!

When arranging work experience, try to think outside the box and realise that there is more to gathering experience than trailing the coat-tails of a harassed doctor all day long. Lots of hospitals require volunteers to befriend and advise patients and their families (see the section on volunteer work below) or even to help deliver the tea. You may even be able to get a paid job in medical records.

You will get a far better insight into the inner workings of hospital life if you spend time there regularly, chatting to patients and staff, rather than sitting in on dull clinics for a couple of days. Your own GP will probably be delighted to let you help out in reception for a couple of days – that will really give you an insight into just how hectic general practice is.

Try to get a variety of experience and explain what you have learnt from it. When I was applying I wrote about how time spent in a GP's surgery made me realise just how crucial teamwork is: if a patient's results get lost in the computer system or not flagged up by the person filing them, then disasters can happen. When I got to interview I was terrified by everyone else recounting stories of their work experience in which they apparently carried out triple heart bypass with a coat hanger while on their lunch break, but actually they had nothing that was worth saying about their experience.

I know you are all honest people, but make sure you are clued up about what you did. One student I interviewed gave an impressive account of some orthopaedic work experience on his statement and then was unable to tell me anything about any of the patients he had seen, which came across rather badly. Always remember that you are demonstrating an understanding of the profession which you can get in lots of different ways: the more unusual your choice of placement, and the more effort you put into analysing what you learnt from it, the better – you want your application to stand out from the crowd.

Volunteer work

Here's an option that is absolutely free, extremely relevant to your future career, teaches you skills that you can put on your personal statement and actually gives something back to the community. If you find that you don't like working with new people, giving your time up for a good cause or sacrificing some of your social life, then you may realise that medicine isn't for you after all. I feel that there is no better way of demonstrating commitment and dedication to a career in the caring professions than actually getting off your bum and helping others. Plus it can be fun. It really doesn't matter what you do – it doesn't even have to be medical or healthcare related.

Getting involved in a project over the medium to long term (i.e. not just a week before you have to write it on your personal statement) can often show more commitment to being a doctor than strutting about in scrubs for a couple of days. Your first port of call if you want to organise some volunteer work is your college careers adviser or community service organiser (a lot of colleges will have them). If you're still at school this might be a little harder, so there are lots of links in the useful contacts section on page 23 to get you started. If nothing here appeals, try looking in your local newspaper or *Yellow Pages*, or you could even pop down to your local school or hospital to see if they need any help with organising fundraising activities.

My top tip is to pick something you think you can stick with for a good period of time, as then you will get the most out of it. There are so many different activities out there, you should be able to find one that doesn't interfere with your school work or part-time job, etc. While you're involved with your chosen activity, keep a few brief notes on the tasks you do and the skills that you develop, and reflect on why it is enjoyable, what is difficult about it and what parts of it you enjoy least. All these thoughts will be vital when it comes to writing your personal statement in order to show what you have learnt from your experience. Additionally, if you get the chance to attend any training courses (such as manual handling, first aid, etc.) as part of your volunteer work, then jump at the opportunity, and it's always a bonus if you can get some sort of written confirmation or certification that you've done it – it's all extra points for your statement.

Academic commitment

In addition to demonstrating your understanding and commitment to a life in medicine, admissions officers also want to see if you will be interested enough to cope with the continued workload while you are at medical school, and whether you have the inquiring mind and natural scientific curiosity desirable in a doctor. You may think that your A-levels are ample demonstration of your commitment to studying, but unfortunately a lot of the competition also has sparkling grades too.

The way that the best students demonstrate their academic enthusiasm and commitment is to read up on an area of science or medicine that interests them. You'll find details in the recommended reading in Chapter 5, but the point here is to start early. The months before your UCAS statement is due in will be filled up with the UKCAT exam, A-level modules and preparation for the BMAT exam, so you won't have that much time for reading then. You can also demonstrate your academic commitment by winning prizes and entering competitions like the Biology and Chemistry Olympiads. In short, make a note of everything you do and read that isn't strictly required for your school or college courses and then it will be easy when you come to write your personal statement.

Extracurricular activities

As if the above requirements weren't proof enough that you are a perfect candidate for medical school, to make your personal statement complete you will have to provide evidence that you are a well rounded individual with plenty of hobbies, interests and enthusiasm for life. In this way, admissions officers will be able to assess whether you have the ability to maintain an appropriate work–life balance which is necessary for your health, happiness and success while at medical school and beyond. Before you ask, there isn't any one thing that really impresses them, so just make sure you get involved in all aspects of life at school or college.

I realise that doing the subjects required for medical school entry doesn't leave you with that much free time, but anything can be used as evidence, from Duke of Edinburgh Awards or football, to playing a musical instrument or being a member of the film society. Try to put yourself forward for positions of responsibility, such as being a school prefect or president of a society. This will show leadership abilities and impress upon them that you are confident and willing to take on duties.

Useful contacts

Work experience and volunteer work

- http://www.volunteering.org.uk/iwantto/ – the Volunteering England website. Contains lots of information and addresses for all sorts of volunteering opportunities.

- www.do-it.org.uk – 'volunteering made easy' – and it really is! Choose what type of project you want to get involved in, where you live and what time you have available, and the database will search through thousands of opportunities to give you a job description and contact details. A fantastic resource.

- www.wwv.org.uk – WorldWide Volunteering website. You can find volunteering opportunities in the UK (free) or anywhere around the world (for which you have to pay £10 to use the search engine), so particularly good for gap-year planning.

Chapter 5
Required reading and other tips for success

This chapter will help you to:

- read around your subject and develop your scientific knowledge
- improve your personal statement
- prepare for your interview.

This chapter is all about preparing yourself so that you can write the best personal statement and perform as well as possible in your interviews, when you get them. You'll be glad to know that I'm not going to recommend that you read the entire Oxford textbook of medicine, nor am I going to insist that you know everything about your life beyond medical school. What I do want you to do is to step up from being an A-level student, where you go to classes, get taught stuff, revise and pass exams, and begin to think like the future doctor you want to be. You need to be spending time reading books and articles instead of watching television, and thinking beyond what you need to know for A-level. Now is the time to start questioning, probing and researching.

In this chapter I have included tips and strategies to help to improve your chances of success. Some of these tips were given to me, some of them I have used with past students. All of them seem to work. With a bit of effort you will find that, not only do they make your application a lot easier, but they will also make life a lot less stressful come interview time.

Read around your subject

To be honest, so far you've probably not been stretched too much at school or college. You turn up, work hard, revise for the exams and get the success you deserve. Unfortunately, there are quite a few of you doing that, and not quite so many places at medical school. So you need something else. Time after time I have sat before grade-A students and asked them what they have read recently (especially as they've just told me how passionate they are about medicine) only to be greeted with a blank look or a defensive 'I've been doing my exams'. What would you say if your interview was tomorrow and you got asked that?

Reading around your subjects indicates interest, enthusiasm, an inquiring mind and dedication, and these seem to be exactly the qualities admissions officers are looking for in medical school applicants. It may sound obvious, and even too simple to be true, but so many students just don't find the time and energy to look beyond their A-level books. An extra bonus is that whatever time you invest in reading around your subject will pay dividends when you come to write the academic part of your personal statement (see Chapter 6) and will also help in your preparation for the BMAT and interview.

You are probably wondering right now what it is that I am going to recommend for you to read. There is only one golden rule here: read something that interests you. It may be something from your studies that you want to go into in greater depth, it may be an article on the news about some new cure for cancer that you thought you'd investigate or it may be a popular-science book that grabbed you in the library. Regarding this last option, you'll find below a list of books either that I read when I was at your stage or that I have had recommended to me by previous students who have enjoyed them. Notice that I said 'enjoyed' – the aim here is development, not punishment.

In contrast with your A-level work, you will probably find that it is actually quite refreshing reading about things that you haven't met before and that provide new concepts that are difficult to grasp. Of course, the list below is by no means exhaustive – feel free to read what you like. These are just examples to get you started. If you find you get particularly interested in a certain topic, enlist the help of a teacher or search the Internet for further reading. Be sure to make notes on any areas of interest so that you can write about them on your personal statement, but only choose topics you would be confident discussing with a potential interviewer.

Recommended reading

- *The Private Life of the Brain* (Susan Greenfield). A riveting read about what goes on inside your skull and what makes us who we are. If you like this, she's written a few more that are worth a read.

- *The Man Who Mistook his Wife for a Hat and other Clinical Tales* (Oliver Sacks). Fascinating. You will actually enjoy reading this one, and it will give you a whole new insight into the interaction between mind and body.

- *Suburban Shaman: Tales from Medicine's Front Line* (Cecil Helman). Gives you a great insight into what life might be like as a doctor. Also thoroughly amusing at times.

- *The Selfish Gene* (Richard Dawkins). You may have seen him on TV. This man has some interesting theories. Just be sure to take them with a pinch of salt – he is rather controversial and not everyone agrees with him.
- *What We Believe but Cannot Prove: Today's Leading Thinkers on Science in the Age of Certainty* (John Brockman, editor). Quite philosophical in parts, but it will definitely get you thinking and, more importantly, questioning everything you read in the future.
- *Nature via Nurture: Genes, Experience and What Makes Us Human* (Matt Ridley). This book is a great read and will set you up nicely for discussions on whether it is our genes or our lifestyles that contribute to health and disease.

Know your medical schools

You may have already decided where you want to apply to read medicine, or you may still be in the process of reading prospectuses and visiting universities. What is critical at this stage is that, once you have decided on your choice of course, you must make sure you know what you're letting yourself in for. For example, it isn't a great idea to let slip at your interview for University A that you much prefer the integrated style of teaching when in fact they pride themselves on the more traditional style of course. Similarly, before you go putting on your personal statement that you are desperate to do an intercalated degree, you had better check that all the medical schools you are applying to offer the chance to do one.

There are over 30 medical schools in the UK that you can apply to, and obviously you aren't going to be extra-knowledgeable about each one, but once you've narrowed the field make sure you request every brochure, leaflet and prospectus you can lay your hands on to find out as much as you can about the course that, hopefully, you will be studying very shortly. Most of the medical schools now have excellent websites that you can browse at your leisure.

When your time comes to go to interview, read up about the course. What attracted you to it? Why study in the area? What do you think are the major health challenges facing the area? (I can promise you, they are very different in central London compared with St Andrews!) What are you looking forward to most about studying at that medical school? Do your research first and it will pay off.

It would be rather nice to get an offer from just one of your choices, but a little flattery goes a long way, and admissions officers who have to sit all day quizzing trembling teenagers will certainly sit up and take notice of someone who's clued up, enthusiastic and thinks that they are working for the best institution in the world. (Note to the wise: you can't fake this type of enthusiasm convincingly, so only apply to places you really want to go to, as opposed to ones where your teacher/mate/postman told you that you'd have a better chance.)

What about your gap year?

I am often asked whether it will affect your application if you decide to have a gap year. The answer is, it depends. Not very helpful advice you may think, but actually the 'depends' bit is dependent on how well you can sell yourself and your plans. On the plus side of having a gap year is that you approach medical school one year older (and hopefully wiser), and that you can bring additional life experience to your studies. On the down side, you are one year further from remembering all that vital stuff you learnt in chemistry, and perhaps you've lost that whole work ethic that was going on while you were at school. So, if you want to have a gap year, you have to prove it's worth the time.

You may be planning to spend your gap year working to earn some cash before university, or you may have plans for travel. Whatever the case, you need to have a clear idea of what it is exactly that you want to do – ideally before your personal statement is submitted and definitely before your interview. It's not good enough to ask for a year out and then think you'll sort it out later. If you are thinking of travelling, it is important to think about where you will go and what you will do during your time. Most importantly, you must set out what you expect to learn from your gap year and how this will help you at medical school.

For example, teaching in an English school in Africa will help you to be independent, will increase your confidence in your verbal and non-verbal communication and will allow you to practise seeking ways around problems. If you say something like this either on your personal statement or in an interview, then they'll probably be waving you off at the quayside with your place on hold until you return. Even if you are working for financial reasons, think about what sort of job you want to get and what you will ideally learn from it.

As long as you can justify the year you will be spending away from medical school, then you won't be penalised. The only point to remember is that, in offering you a deferred place, they are theoretically denying a person in the year below you a place. If you are only an average candidate they may be unwilling to take the gamble that someone better won't come along next year. However, if you are a strong candidate anyway, then they'll be more than happy to accommodate you and your year out.

There *is* a life after medical school

If you have a doctor in the family or a sibling at medical school, then you may have some idea as to what will happen when you skip out of medical school clutching your hard-earned degree. If not, you may be rather bewildered and worried at the stories that have been doing the rounds about students coming out of medical school with no job to go to, or being unable to find work in the area of their choice.

The truth is that the whole process of recruiting and training junior doctors is undergoing a huge reshuffle, under the title of Modernising Medical Careers (MMC). In short, once you emerge from medical school, you will enter a two-year 'foundation programme' which is equivalent to the old pre-registration house-officer year and the first senior house-officer year. Once these are completed, you can enter specialty training or do general training if you are still not sure what specialty is right for you.

It is well worth having a look at the website www.mmc.nhs.uk and spending some time familiarising yourself with the basics of it all. Also on the website are some excellent case studies of different specialties, which are really useful to clue you up on what you need to do and how long it will all take. Don't worry yourself too much about all the details – you aren't going to get the Spanish Inquisition on it at interview, not least because the whole system is in a state of flux at the moment. I would suggest it is worth knowing a little about it, though, especially as it will directly affect you in the not too distant future.

In short, the best way to prepare yourself for your application to medical school is to treat it like preparing for a job interview. You should research the company's position, its ethos, its strengths and its weaknesses. You should find out about your career pathway and demonstrate that you have the skills and the commitment required to succeed in a competitive arena. Most importantly, come the time of the interview, you need to convince the company (or medical school) that, if they fail to hire you, they will be missing out on the best candidate for the job by far. Think like a professional and, hopefully, you'll hear those wonderful words: 'You're hired!'

Chapter 6
How to write the perfect personal statement

This chapter will help you to:

■ understand the purpose of your personal statement

■ plan your personal statement

■ produce a polished, effective personal statement.

It is a fact universally acknowledged that someone who finds it easy to write 700 words in praise of him or herself is probably in need of a good slap. I clearly remember the sheer horror of staring at a blank computer screen and realising that, within a few days, I would have to produce what has probably been the most important document I have ever written in my life. I say this not to scare you but to impress upon you that, just as Rome wasn't built in a day, your personal statement will take a bit longer than your bus journey to school or college on the day of the deadline.

In this chapter we will consider briefly what the point of a personal statement is, what it should include (and what it shouldn't) and, most importantly, how you can make your own personal statement so brilliant that you will be utterly irresistible to medical school admissions officers everywhere.

What is the point of a personal statement?

Your teachers have told you that it's important, your friends are worrying about theirs already and even the UCAS application form online allows you to write and rewrite your statement until you're heartily sick of it. But just why is the statement so important, especially now that you are being assessed in so many other ways, such as the UKCAT and BMAT?

Your personal statement works in two ways. First, the admissions officers who have to trudge through the thousands of applications that land on their desk need something to differentiate Miss A, who has six A grades at A1 and is described by her teachers as 'truly and utterly a wonderful student', from Mr B, who also has six grade As and whose teachers 'couldn't carry on living without him'. Similarly, they want to know if Miss A has actually done anything but study during her years at school, and need to understand the rationale behind Mr B's decision to take a year out.

Secondly, the personal statement gives you a chance to show why you are so ideally suited to a career in medicine rather than law, accountancy or investment banking, and why, if given the chance, you would make more of your place at medical school than the people left behind on the pile.

The critical point is this: if you are applying to medicine you are bright. All of you could, without a doubt, pass your exams at medical school and, with a bit of work, go on to be a competent doctor. But the medical schools don't just want students who are going to pass their exams with the bare minimum of work; nor do they want to produce doctors who are one-dimensional and have vitamin D deficiency from never emerging from the library. The doctors of the future have to have the drive to succeed, the passion to put themselves forward for challenges and the humanity to realise when they have made mistakes and to assess their own limitations. The only real way that admissions officers can assess if you fit these criteria is if you tell them that you do in your personal statement. If you don't put it in, then they'll assume you aren't what they are looking for and pass you by.

Approaching your statement

The first thing to do is to start early. Your statement has to be in to UCAS by the middle of October, and your teachers will probably want to sit on it (or 'check it') for a month before that, which means you probably want to be putting the finishing touches to your statement around the beginning of September (I promise you, it will be such a nice feeling when it's finished). So I would advise starting to write your statement around August. Of course, as this is the summer holidays, there is plenty of preparation that you can do beforehand in order to make the writing whiz by when you have to sit down to do it.

The advice below has resulted from my experience over a number of years helping many students with their statements, and it really seems to work. Whether you are starting to think about your statement a year in advance or are panicking a week before it is due in, following the outline below will enable you to organise your statement in a logical and involving way.

Start with an empty sheet of A4 paper and divide it into three equal sections (see Figure 1). The first section is entitled 'Academic basis of medicine' (this is explained below), the second 'Experience and understanding' and the third 'Skills of a doctor'. Leave a small space at the top and bottom – these will eventually become your introduction and conclusion, which we'll leave to the very last as this is probably the hardest bit.

If you are starting to think about your personal statement early, then this page will be rather empty but, as you get involved with extracurricular activities, complete work experience or volunteer work and read journals and books, remember to jot each example down, and then by the time you come to write your statement it will be a piece of cake. For the rest of you who have slightly less time, you are going to have to sit down and rack your brains for examples to go in these boxes. At this stage just jot down brief notes and examples; you can work on each section in more detail later.

Figure 1 Approaching your statement

Academic basis of medicine
Experience and understanding (work experience)
Skills of a doctor (extracurricular)

Academic basis of medicine

Medicine is probably unique among the professions in that you will never stop learning until the day you retire. Despite what a lot of consultants might say about themselves, you will never know everything, and what you do know will be constantly proved wrong. Fifty years ago, medical students hadn't even heard of subjects like gene-technology and sociology – today they form a large part of the curriculum. So you can bet that, within your lifetime, you'll be struggling to come to terms with new ideas too.

To cope with these new ideas, the doctors of tomorrow have to be able to demonstrate that they are interested in science, understand the ideals behind evidence-based medicine and actually enjoy studying. This is the section in which you get the chance to demonstrate your thirst for knowledge and your genuine interest in medicine as a science (and you'd better be interested now, because you're sure as anything going to have moments where you are mightily sick of it all during medical school!).

A lot of medical schools these days make a big fuss over their 'integrated' courses (problem-based learning, patients from day one and so on). The truth of the matter is that you can't run before you can crawl, and you aren't going to be diagnosing Mrs Jones' haemorrhoids before you know your basic anatomy, biochemistry and pharmacology. So you had better like studying! They want students who are dedicated enough to be up all night studying even when there isn't an exam the next morning.

You have a lot of work on your plate with your A1 and A2 courses, but it's not much of an effort to read around a subject that interests you or to read a 'pop' science book (see Chapter 5). I have lost count of the times I have seen in a statement, 'I regularly read the *New Scientist*'. Even if you do read it, is it really that impressive?

In order to impress, you have to get specific. When I was at your stage, I was really interested in Alzheimer's disease. I went down to my local library and got out a selection of books, from self-help books for carers of people with the disease to a small science book with theories of how the disease affects the brain. I wrote about this on my personal statement, and in my interview I was asked about it. We had a really interesting discussion about the topic, and I was asked lots of scientific questions about protein structure as a related topic. I think that they must have realised I was interested and motivated enough to get off the sofa and read around a topic of my choice and, although looking back I knew absolutely nothing of the importance of the disease itself, this is what counted and I got the place. The point of this is to show you that there are ways you can *prove* your academic dedication, rather than just talking about it.

Important note: they don't care particularly which books/articles you read, and they definitely won't be testing you on their contents, so please don't become obsessed about reading lots of important-looking medical textbooks (there's lots of time for you to do that once you're at medical school). Also, never, ever, ever put a book or article on your statement that you are intending to read: you might not get around to it, and you will look like an idiot at interview trying to explain just why exactly you didn't make the time to read it (I have seen this happen).

Read something you are actually interested in so that your enthusiasm will shine through. Perhaps it's something you have been studying at school, like genetics, or perhaps a friend or relative has a disease like diabetes that you wanted to know more about. I'm not that old, but in my day we had to use libraries to find out information. Life is much easier now: pop any old search term into a search engine and you will come up with thousands of sites describing your chosen topic (although stay away from eBay – I doubt you can buy 'everything to do with "Cloning" items' there … try it!).

While you are reading, think about how these 'facts' have been found out – just because it is in a book doesn't mean it's true. If you do this you will start to develop the critical appraisal skills you will use throughout your career. For example, how do we know that HIV causes AIDS? How do they go about developing the new 'wonder-drugs' that are always on the news? You should be able to find a topic out there that interests you; just make sure you read something in addition to your necessary school or college work – it looks so bad if you show no evidence of an interest in the scientific world. Whatever it is, write about it in your statement (see the examples in Box 1), and be ready to talk about it at interview.

Box 1 Reading round: examples

I have been enjoying my A1 biology module on genetics, and I developed a particular interest in cystic fibrosis. During Internet searches I came across a number of theories regarding why the disease allele is so prevalent in the Caucasian population, including one which described a possible link between the allele carrier state and resistance against cholera, similar to the possible link between sickle-cell carrier status and malaria resistance which I have already studied. However, I have been unable to find any evidence for this theory, which has taught me that, however appealing an idea may be, it is important to realise that it is only a theory unless proven.

During my voluntary work at a nursing home I realised I knew very little about diseases of mental health. I have since read The Man Who Mistook his Wife for a Hat, by Oliver Sacks, which has given me an insight into the complexity of the human brain and made me appreciate the importance of recognising and promoting mental health issues. This reading has given me a new insight into caring for the residents in the nursing home, and has helped me to deal with my own concerns and feelings about mental health.

After reading a newspaper article about the growing epidemic of obesity in the UK, I have been reading about the different measures being taken to reverse the problem, including public health measures, education and drug treatments. During my research I came across a study in which a gene knockout mouse became extremely obese, which led to a possibility that this gene could be missing in people who overeat. However, I found out this was not the case, and in discussions with my teacher I have explored the impact of social and psychological factors involved in diet, which has made me appreciate that disease does not always have a cause-and-effect relationship.

Also in this section you can write about any prizes you have won that demonstrate how much you love science and studying it. For example, you may have won the chemistry prize at school, or received a certificate for taking part in the Biology Olympiad. They may not seem incredibly exciting to you, but if you don't put it in then they can't judge its worth.

Rather than just listing your achievements, try to weave them into a sentence demonstrating your skills so that the award or prize becomes proof that you have such abilities. For example: 'During the last term I have been working hard to improve my laboratory skills, particularly in the areas of planning and precision. This work has been recognised through the award of the ICI Challenge Trophy in Chemistry, which I was delighted to win.'

Once you get started you will probably find that you have quite a few examples, so choose your best ones and try to formulate them into sentences so that the academic basis of medicine statement takes up about one third of your 4,000 available characters. You'll probably find that, at this stage, it is easier to use the computer so that you can play about with words and sentences (but go easy on the thesaurus – it often stands out like a sore thumb when you've been over-using it!). At this stage also, don't worry about getting the section into final draft form; this is best done at the end when you bring all the sections together.

Experience and understanding

This is the place to put down all the work experience and voluntary work you have been doing over the past years or months (see Chapter 4 for more detail about this, and for what to do if you've left it all a bit late). Medical schools are looking for students who have demonstrated their commitment to medicine and who understand what the job is about, and the demands that will be placed upon them. I always think that this is a bit of an unfair expectation, seeing as even now I don't really know what's going to hit me when I start work. Also, they keep on changing the arrangements for junior doctors so that the NHS when you start may be very different from the one today. But in theory it's a good idea, and seeing as you want to spend the next 10–15 years of your life in training for a profession, you may as well know what you are letting yourself in for!

However, it is this section that probably causes the most anxiety among applicants. Some of you may find it easy to arrange places and so have a wealth of experiences to draw upon when writing your statement. Others of you may not have a friendly orthopaedic surgeon in your back pocket and so are feeling rather ashamed of your two weeks' filing in your local GP's surgery, or voluntary work in the care home down the road. Again, the lesson here is not what you have done, but what you have learnt from it.

If, during your time with the orthopaedic surgeon, you sat yawning while he saw patient after patient, then you haven't really had any insight into a career in medicine. If, however, you went and talked to one of the old ladies who was having a knee replacement and asked her about why she was having it done, and then asked the surgeon why she had to wait so long for it, you probably will have more insight into the health service than most medical students.

A lot of students also want to use this section to describe what sort of job they want to go into, be it general practitioner or cardiologist. My advice here is to proceed with caution: unless you have always desperately wanted to do it and it has been your *raison d'être* for going into medicine, then I would save the space and not bother – everyone changes his or her mind about 20 times during the course of medical school, so it's neither here nor there.

To make life easier for yourself, split this section of your page into three (see Box 2), and fill in the work experience and voluntary work you have done. For each example, write what you did, what you have learnt and why it is important to your future career. Always think whether you would give a place to yourself based on what you are writing. If you wouldn't, then it's probably not convincing enough. Again, always be honest – you'll find you have lots of good examples if you just think about them for a while. I've included a few examples to get you going.

Box 2 Experience and understanding

What I did	What I did or learnt	Why is it important?
Two weeks in a GP's surgery	Filing patient records Observed consultations	Importance of good note-keeping Stresses of general practice How important the non-medical staff at the practice are How computers are so important in the NHS
One year nursing home (once a week)	Chatted to residents Chatted to residents' families Delivered medicines	How to communicate with different sections of society Elderly people are reluctant to complain – need to ask if there are problems Problems with taking lots of different medicines
One week chest unit at local hospital	Attended ward round Sat in on clinic Talked to patients	How medical team works Importance of physio/occupational therapy Patient distress at uncertainty

Once you have done this, transfer your work to the computer to start formulating your examples into prose. So with the final example in Box 2, the week at the chest unit, you could write something similar to that shown in Box 3.

Box 3 Work experience

In order to gain a better appreciation of what life as a junior doctor would be like, I spent a week shadowing various members of the COPD treatment team at Getwellsoon General Hospital. Attending ward rounds allowed me to understand how important good team dynamics are in formulating treatment and management plans, and I was surprised to see that physiotherapy and occupational therapy were more often used in treatment plans than I had previously thought. Talking to patients in the clinics made me realise that uncertainty about diagnoses and worries about serious illness contribute greatly to their anxiety, and I observed how the consultant spent a lot of time talking to his patients to alleviate this.

Anyone reading an example like this would get a real flavour for what you did during your time there (which immediately banishes any doubts that you made it up), and that you learnt something from your experience. Don't be afraid of describing operations you saw or a patient you talked to/followed up. Just be sure to remove his or her details. It all helps to make your statement more vivid and memorable.

Skills of a doctor

The thing that continues to surprise and delight me about the students of today is that you seem to have an endless capacity for extracurricular activities: from the Duke of Edinburgh Award to a seat on the student United Nations council, from world chess champions to awards for gymnastics. However, these incredible achievements can literally count for nothing if you neglect to present them in the right way. The admissions officers don't work on a points system which gives, say, eight points for being world indoor tiddlywinks champion and three points for duck-feeding duties at the local pond-life club. What they are looking for is evidence that you have a good work–life balance and have constantly sought out challenges to develop and stretch yourself.

So, if you take one thing away from this chapter, then take this: for every achievement you describe on your form, you must say 1) what it meant to you; and 2) what you have learnt from it. If you do this I can promise that your statement will far surpass 95 per cent of the other statements in the pile. Have a look at some of the 'before' and 'after' examples in Box 4 to get a feel for what I mean. They may sound cheesy at first read, but just imagine how refreshing it is for an admissions officer who has already seen 500 forms to read one that spells out for him or her exactly how hard you worked for your Duke of Edinburgh Gold award and how achieving it has given you a whole new take on teamwork – not to mention how useful these skills will be once you're at medical school!

Box 4 Personal achievements: examples

Before

I am working towards my Duke of Edinburgh Gold Award and we are planning to go hiking in the Peak District. This has taught me lots of teamwork skills.

(They think: Everyone's doing Duke of Edinburgh, no proof of achievement, no evidence of teamwork skills.)

After

During my Duke of Edinburgh Silver trip in the Vale of Glamorgan my team ran short of provisions. As a result I have assumed responsibility for food and water for our upcoming Gold Award trip to the Peak District. I have developed a spreadsheet which details our precise requirements and I am confident that my organisation will enable the team to perform at its peak during the challenge.

(They think: Not afraid of responsibility, organised, team-player.)

Before

Last summer I went to the student United Nations conference on HIV-AIDS. We attended lots of lectures and I produced a report about the problem of HIV in Africa.

(They think: Very passive, no real show of interest in the subject.)

After

As a delegate at the student United Nations summit on AIDS I produced a report about the problem of HIV in Africa. During my research I had to develop the skills of critical appraisal and became aware of the problems of using second-hand evidence. I was very moved by the scale of the disaster in Africa and elsewhere and have since completed a charity run in aid of the Terence Higgins Foundation.

(They think: Wow! Evidence of new skills being learnt and personal involvement in the project.)

Before

In my spare time I play the position of striker in the college second football team. This demonstrates teamwork and also leadership skills as I have to motivate my team to score goals. We won the cup this year, which was a great personal achievement for me.

(They think: Some attempt to show what has been learnt, but no real evidence: rather generic.)

After

My position of striker in the college second team has impressed upon me the importance of teamwork. In the cup final this year we suffered a number of injuries and I decided to substitute myself in order to bring defence players on. Although disappointed not to be playing, it paid off as we narrowly won. The time commitment needed to play has been a challenge with my college work, but has helped me to develop the organisation and flexibility that will be required in my future studies.

(They think: Evidence of teamwork and organisation. I really feel like I know this candidate.)

Bear in mind that it isn't what you have done that is important, but rather what you have learnt from it and how it has helped you develop as a person now and how this will impact on your suitability to be a medical student and future doctor. A lot of people feel they have to lie or 'stretch the truth' in their statements because they feel a place in the second netball team is inadequate, or painting the scenery in the drama show doesn't demonstrate enough flair. With careful consideration of what you have learnt from each activity plus a well phrased explanation of why it was important to you that you were involved/achieved your aim, even the most basic of activities becomes an excellent example of your suitability for a career in medicine.

I have read many personal statements in my time and often the ones that, in theory, should be the most impressive read like a dull list of someone else's achievements (which isn't really ever interesting to anyone but yourself and your proud parents!). The statements that are always the most impressive are the ones from students who perhaps haven't had the opportunity or ability to participate in a huge variety of top-notch activities, but have made sure that they have given their all to the ones they have been involved in and learnt a lot as a result. So the next time you're halfway up a mountain or scoring a hockey penalty, think about why you're doing it and what skills you are developing. It's quite hard at first but you'll soon get used to it and it will make for an excellent personal statement.

If you're stuck about what sort of qualities you need to demonstrate, think about what qualities you would want in a doctor who was treating you for a broken leg. You'd want knowledge and skills as standard, but then how about good communication skills, and interpersonal skills? You'd also need stamina to treat a waiting room full of patients, but dedication enough to treat each one as if he or she were the first. If you then think of an example when you demonstrated your skills, you'll be well on your way to some great examples and you will make life so much easier for the admissions officers who are looking for these very same attributes.

Introduction and conclusion

I've left this until last as it's often the most difficult part to get right, and now you're over your writers' block it should be a lot easier. A good introduction and conclusion are vital, both to catch and hold the attention and to summarise your statement concisely.

Bad examples of what to write for an introduction include 'since my sister fell over when she was two and knocked her tooth out I knew I wanted to be a doctor', and including random statements out of books. These do make your statement stand out, but only for being stupid. If you have had a long-held ambition to study medicine, then that is fine, but try to think about why you want to do it and then use this as your statement opener. For example, 'For me, a career in medicine will allow me to explore my love of science in an arena full of challenges and surprises' is infinitely better than 'I have always wanted to study medicine as I feel it would be the ideal career for someone who loves science and people' because the first example is much more personal.

The conclusion will reflect this opening introduction and will remind the reader that you have demonstrated the skills and attributes required for a place. This is no place for being shy – we need one final fanfare on the trumpet to clinch the deal. A good example might be: 'Through my extracurricular activities and achievements I feel that I have demonstrated the skills and characteristics necessary for a career in the challenging profession of medicine. I hope to continue my personal and academic development at medical school and throughout my future career.'

Putting your statement together

You have just 4,000 characters to play with on the online 'apply' form for UCAS. But at least you have a character counter on your word-processor, so you should have no problem with this. Only transfer it over to the application form when you're happy to submit it. I have heard stories of people pressing the wrong button and a half-finished form being saved! If you've followed the advice above you probably have too many words to fit on, so go through it and be ruthless: cull anything that doesn't scream 'perfect'! You also need to play around with the sentences so that they don't all start with 'I have, I do', etc.

When you have finished with your statement, your teacher will obviously want to see it. Listen to his or her advice, but if you really want to keep something in and you teacher wants you to change it, then stick to your guns. It's your personal statement after all, and too much meddling can take you away from what you want people to see of you.

Important note: if you are applying for other courses other than medicine (for example, your two additional 'insurance courses'), then don't worry about trying to incorporate aptitude for these into your statement. If you're going to go for a medical school place, go for it good and proper, and don't compromise. There will be enough about your love of science and incredible personal achievements in your statement already to satisfy even the most stringent biochemistry or pharmacology degree, and they appreciate and understand the situation that you are put in, so don't worry about it.

Finally, however perfect your statement is it won't look too good with spelling and grammar mistakes, so avail yourself of a spellchecker. But please be aware that it has a habit of changing medical terms into something completely unrecognisable!

After all that work you should have a personal statement to be proud of. Just make sure you save it properly. Save it in at least two separate places, such as a removable disk and your computer area at school or college. Every year computer failures scupper statements a week before due date and you don't need that kind of hassle. As it is very common for interviewers to use a copy of your personal statement as a springboard for discussion at interview, always keep a copy of your statement to revise from the night before. Also make sure you keep all the notes that you have made about your work experience and reading as these will come in very handy to refresh your memory just before your interview.

Chapter 7
Exams and interviews

This chapter will help you to:

■ understand which medical school entry exams you are required to take, and why
■ prepare for your medical school interview.

Exams and interviews are probably the two most horrid things in life, other than haemorrhoids. Once upon a time your A-levels would have been enough to satisfy even the most stringent of admission committees but, unfortunately, we now live in the age of assessment, and if you want to go to medical school you're going to be assessed up to your armpits.

In this chapter you will find all the general and administrative information regarding the UK Clinical Aptitude Test (UKCAT) and the Biomedical Admissions Test (BMAT), and in the second and third parts of this book you will find all the materials you need to practise the types of question that will come up in these exams until you're satisfied you've become an expert. After all that practice you'll surely get a fantastic mark and lots of interview offers, and so the final part of this chapter looks at some dos and don'ts at interview and how you can prepare for success.

All about the UKCAT

Introduced in 2006, the UKCAT is an aptitude test designed to assess whether or not you have the appropriate professional attitude, mental abilities and problem-solving skills that will be necessary for a successful career in medicine or dentistry. It's used by a selection of medical schools as part of the application procedure (i.e. they look at your personal statement, your predicted grades and your teacher reference too) and they may use it to help to decide whether to call you for interview or offer you a place. The following medical and dental courses require you to sit the UKCAT as part of your application:

University of Aberdeen	A100
Brighton and Sussex Medical School	A100
Cardiff University	A100, A104, A200, A204
University of Dundee	A100, A104, A200, A204
University of Durham	A106
University of East Anglia	A100

University of Edinburgh	A100, A104
University of Glasgow	A100, A200
Hull York Medical School	A100
Keele University	A100
King's College London	A100, A101, A102, A103, A202, A203, A205
Imperial College London Graduate	A101
University of Leeds	A100
University of Leicester	A100, A101
University of Manchester	A104, A106, A204, A206
University of Newcastle upon Tyne	A101, A106, A206
University of Nottingham	A100
University of Oxford Graduate Entry Medical Degree	A101
Peninsula Medical School	A100
Queen Mary, University of London	A100, A101, A200, A201
Queen's University, Belfast	A100, A200
University of Sheffield	A100, A104, A200
University of Southampton	A100, A102
University of St Andrews	A100
St George's, University of London	A100
Warwick University Gradute Entry	A101

So, as you can see from all the universities that require it, you're probably going to have to sit the UKCAT. The need for the UKCAT has arisen mainly out of the continuing increase in immensely well qualified applicants for medicine, leaving admissions officers with little to distinguish one candidate from another. The UKCAT does not include any questions that require science or A-level knowledge: think of it like an IQ or mental ability test. However, like anything in life, practice makes perfect, and you'll probably want to practise the types of questions likely to come up. You can look at the ones on the website (www.ukcat.ac.uk) and also use all the ones in this book.

In terms of the test administration, all the details can be found on the website, but in brief you will have to register online to take the test during or after June, and you can sit the test anytime you like before the deadline, which is 10 October 2008. You will have to pay £60 (£95 for overseas students) to take the test, although bursaries will be available for those in financial need (make sure you apply via the website before you register to sit the test).

You will sit the test at a registered centre using a computer, and in total it will take around two hours. Results are available immediately, in theory enabling you to take your result into consideration before you have to submit your UCAS application form. However – there is no clear guidance available as to what constitutes a 'good' score – so, I would consider it wise to see your result as part of your assessment and continue with your application to medical or dental school whatever the result.

All about the BMAT

The BMAT is a little older and wiser than its cousin, the UKCAT. It has been around for a number of years and is required for students applying to the medicine, veterinary medicine and related courses listed below:

University of Cambridge	A100, A101, D100
Imperial College London (University of London)	A100
University of Oxford Medical School	A100 B100
Royal Veterinary College	D100, D101
University College London	A100

The BMAT consists of three sections, and it is a paper exam sat at your school or college or local test centre. You'll sit this in early November, so it shouldn't clash with the UKCAT. The first paper tests problem-solving and analysing arguments; the second tests your science and maths knowledge; and the third tests your ability to create structured, coherent arguments in an essay format. All the information you need regarding the test, including practice papers, sample answers and arrangements for sitting the test, is available on the BMAT website (www.bmat.org.uk), which should be your first point of call for all your test queries.

I personally think that there's a lot you can do to prepare for the BMAT, which is why you will find a detailed section later in this book telling you just how to approach the questions and with lots of examples for you to practise. Before the UKCAT came along, students used to get very stressed over the idea of the BMAT, but now you have the UKCAT to worry about too.

Oxford, Cambridge, UCL and Imperial all have a reputation among students as being 'hard' to get into, and by allowing themselves to have a different test from all the other medical schools, they probably haven't helped their cause any. But the BMAT is a sensible test once you get the hang of it, and so don't let it put you off applying to those universities.

Time management for the BMAT and UKCAT

By reading this book you will begin to understand the style and scope of the UKCAT and BMAT examination questions, and will hopefully realise that most of the questions do not present an intellectual challenge greater than that of your A-level courses. This is not to say that the exams are a walk-over: the difficulty of these tests comes from the fact that the time allowed for their completion is extremely short, and that each of the subtests is individually timed and scored, preventing you from making up for lost time in areas of the test which you find easier. Until you have taken some mock examinations you won't really appreciate how difficult it is to answer all of the questions in the time available, and you certainly won't have much time (if any) for checking your answers. So throughout your preparation for the UKCAT and BMAT you need to focus on working accurately under time pressure and improving your performance in your weakest parts of the papers. Every year, even the most diligent students emerge from the examination room feeling that the exam was more difficult than they had expected and anxious that they didn't manage to complete or check all of their answers to the best of their ability. This is the challenge of the UKCAT and BMAT exams, and it is helpful to think of this situation as a mark of a successful examination method rather than a failure of the candidate. After all, there isn't much point taking an extra examination if there is no scope for stretching the very best students.

Below are a number of suggestions to help you to prepare yourself for the time pressure you will encounter in the UKCAT and BMAT examinations; as always, adequate preparations and practice will help to increase your confidence and alleviate much of the anxiety and stress of the exams.

Attempt practice papers with 10 per cent less time allowance

It is much less stressful doing a practice paper sat in your bedroom with the cat in your lap and a plate of chocolate digestives within reach than it is doing the real thing in a cold school assembly hall with 40 other stressed-out candidates. To allow for in this panic factor always give yourself 10 per cent less time when you are doing the practice papers than you will be allowed for the real thing: hopefully by the time you get to the real exam you will be so efficient that you can use this 'free time' for checking or re-attempting tricky questions.

Attempt the practice papers 'blind'

Often it is tempting to have a look through the practice papers before you actually have a go at them: if you do this then your brain becomes familiar with the problems and may even start to subconsciously solve them before you actually come to sit the paper, hence the time pressure feels less acute. In short, it is easy to answer a question once you have seen it before (and may even have half glanced at the answer while looking at another solution).

Have an order

The biggest cause of panic for most students is turning over the paper and feeling they can't answer the first question, or the second, or the fifth, tenth, etc. This triggers a spiral of panic which can be extremely costly timewise. Having a set order to how you tackle the paper really assists in helping you to achieve a sense of control. Whether you attempt the questions in the order they come, take the biology questions first in the BMAT or tackle the hardest/longest ones first/last in the UKCAT, always keep this same order when practising sample papers and then you won't feel so phased in the exam room when you come across a tough first question.

Become a confident guesser

No negative marking on the BMAT and UKCAT means that even if you haven't a clue as to the answer, then you have approximately a 20 per cent chance of getting it right. That means, in a trade-off between spending the dying seconds of the exam trying to work out a complex bit of algebra, or answering an easy question and guessing a hard one, then it's worth a guess every time. This feels very strange for students used to carefully working out each answer, but the exams are constructed so as to allow for intelligent guesswork. This is something that you can practise with sample papers: never look up the answer to a question you can't do until you've made a guess at it – you will find in time that you develop a sixth sense for canny guesses.

Courses not requiring tests

Some of you may have noticed that there are a few medical schools offering standard entry courses that require neither the BMAT nor the UKCAT. These are the University of Bristol and the University of Liverpool. There may be some among you hatching a plan for an application that requires no tests by applying to these two medical schools. I wouldn't advise you to go down that route, mainly because these medical schools are likely to have lots of people applying to them as an 'insurance' place in case they fail the UKCAT, and so they may already be extra-competitive to get into. Additionally, there isn't much point in applying to a medical school you don't particularly want to go to merely to avoid a test which, with a bit of work, you can ace anyway.

Instead of thinking about the tests as a negative part of your application, look at them as having the potential to help you. The very fact you own this book indicates that you are committed to lots of hard work and preparation for the BMAT/UKCAT. If this is the case, then your test result will actually give you an advantage over everyone else, rather than it hampering your application. Just be sure to follow the advice and to practise the questions in the second and third parts of this book.

Interviews

Interviews are funny things. You spend the months that follow the submission of your UCAS form hoping, dreaming and praying that you'll get an interview. Then, when you get an interview, you're sent flying into a mad panic because you're not prepared, you don't know what they're going to ask you and, most importantly, you don't know what to wear.

Many interviews take the form of a friendly discussion or chat with a member of the medical school staff and/or a clinical doctor. They'll want to know a bit about you, find out how interested you are in the subject and see whether you have the type of mind that they could teach easily (i.e. open to new ideas, able to think your way around problems). Hopefully, you followed all the previous advice regarding extra reading and voluntary work, and so you're going to have plenty to talk about at interview. If not, you can put in a week or so of hard work reading the medical sections of the newspapers and thinking about some answers to ethical problems, such as euthanasia, abortion, premature babies, etc. (for more on this, see the section on the BMAT exam). Then, when they ask you, 'What have you been reading lately?' you won't sit there dumbstruck or say 'the back of the shampoo bottle' (yes, someone really did say this… luckily it was a mock interview!).

Remember that anything on your personal statement is fair game for an interview topic, so make sure that you keep a copy of it to refresh your memory before your interview. They may use it to spark off a conversation with you about your reading or work experience so, to repeat my advice, you should only put on items that you are comfortable talking about.

If they ask you about an ethical problem treat it like an essay and always explore the ideas behind both sides of the debate – this will really impress them and demonstrate your mature and non-judgemental nature. Throwing in a few relevant examples from your reading and topical awareness will also make you appear more committed so, if you know something about a particular topic, don't be afraid to share it. Also, don't be afraid to disagree with the interviewer if you have a valid reason for doing so. As long as you always back up your argument, you'll be fine, and they'll probably give you extra respect marks for sticking to your guns.

The number-one worry that students have is that they don't have a perfect answer to the dreaded question, 'So, young person, why do you want to be a doctor?' I was never asked this during my interviews, but some people are asked it, generally to break the ice and because the interviewers are not a particularly original bunch. Remember, there is no A* answer: your enthusiasm is more important than a lot of waffle you rehearsed in advance. Just give your real reasons and, if they don't make the interviewers run for the straitjacket, then they're perfect.

When it comes to choosing your wardrobe for the interview, think conservative. You don't have to wear a suit, but you shouldn't go for the 'Saturday-night-on-the-town' look either. Doctors in hospitals no longer wear jackets (for infection control reasons), and some don't even wear ties, so don't feel you have to dress up. Imagine that you are a patient and you are interviewing a prospective doctor who is going to perform some very intimate surgery on you: what sort of image would you like him or her to portray through his or her clothes and appearance? If the image doesn't say 'ripped jeans', then they're probably best left at home. It's the same with hair (facial and otherwise): think smart, clean and tidy.

Finally, I always hear people talking about things the interviewers will do to 'psyche you out', like whistling or reading a book. If they do happen to do these things (and I doubt they ever would), it's because they're rather rude, as opposed to some dastardly plan to test you out. The interviewers really are there to try to find the best in you: they have to fill up their medical school with the best people they can find, so it's in no one's interest if you are so terrified you can hardly speak. The biggest challenge is to become comfortable talking about yourself. You are practising your interview technique when you are talking about your interests and your reading with your friends and family, so it shouldn't feel so weird and big headed when you're sitting in your interview and have to start chatting away about similar things.

When you come out of any exam or interview, bear in mind that your brain is wired up to remind you only of the questions that you got wrong, or the idiotic things that you said in the heat of the moment. Try to forget about these, and think of everything as a learning experience. You'll know the result soon enough and, in the meantime, you deserve a pat on the back for all your hard work.

Looking to the future

If you win a place at one of the medical schools of your choice, throw yourself a big party and then make sure you work hard enough to get your A-levels (it would be silly to throw your place away after all that hard work, but every year this happens). If you haven't been so lucky, then don't despair: if you want to take up a place on your non-medical degree course, then make sure you get the required grades. There is always the possibility of getting into medicine via the graduate route after you have completed your degree. Some students decide they are still determined to study medicine and take a year out to reapply. Whatever you decide, make sure you talk over all the options thoroughly with your teachers, parents and careers adviser: you have the rest of your life either to applaud or regret your decision, so it doesn't have to be made quickly.

Part II
Preparing for the UK Clinical Aptitude Test (UKCAT)

This part of the book will help you to:

- understand the purpose and the format of the UK Clinical Aptitude Test (UKCAT)
- understand the format and design of multiple-choice questions
- understand the different elements of the UKCAT and how to tackle them
- prepare for the test using appropriate aptitude and reasoning questions.

Introduction

The UK Clinical Aptitude Test (UKCAT) was introduced for use in the selection process by a consortium of UK universities' medical and dental schools. The 26 universities comprising the consortium and the courses requiring applicants to sit the UKCAT are listed in Chapter 7. The test will be used in 2008 for both entry to the universities in 2009 and deferred entry for 2010.

As with the BioMedical Admissions Test (BMAT), or other entry examination requirements, this test is designed to help universities to make more informed choices among the many highly qualified applicants who apply for medical and dental degree programmes. The test has apparently been designed to assess those skills, traits and behaviours that identify individuals who will be successful in clinical careers.

The UKCAT is an onscreen examination and comprises five subtests: Verbal Reasoning, Quantitative Reasoning, Abstract Reasoning, Decision Analysis and Non-Cognitive Analysis. Each of these subtests will be in a multiple-choice format and timed separately. The overall examination is to be delivered in two hours.

There are two versions of the UKCAT: the standard UKCATand UKCATSEN (Special Educational Needs). The UKCATSEN is a longer version of the UKCAT intended for candidates that require special arrangements due to a documented medical condition or with disabilities.

According to Pearson VUE, the test designers, 'The test will not contain any curriculum nor any science content; nor can it be revised for. It will focus on exploring the cognitive powers of candidates and other attributes considered to be valuable to health care professionals.' However, the types of test being presented by Pearson VUE have been in existence for many decades and are used widely in the selection, assessment and development of staff. None of these commercially available tests claims to have a curriculum content and cannot specifically be revised for. However, it has been demonstrated that practising such tests does increase both levels of competence and performance. It also helps to reduce anxiety levels in that applicants are not faced with the unknown.

For those of you who are 'fortunate' enough to be sitting both the UKCAT and BMAT, there is some overlap in the areas being assessed. The BMAT has three sections: Aptitude and Skills, Scientific Knowledge and Application, and a Writing Task. The Aptitude and Skills section includes three separate tests: problem-solving, understanding argument, and data analysis and influence. The problem-solving element contains some numerical-type multi-choice questions that are of a similar format to those in the UKCAT Quantitative Reasoning subtest. There are also some numerical-type questions within the Scientific Knowledge and Application section of the BMAT. In relation to understanding argument, this may also have some parallels with the UKCAT Verbal Reasoning subtest.

Format and design of multiple-choice questions

This section provides a brief overview of multiple-choice question tests and then examines their format and design and, in particular, the design being suggested for use in the UKCAT.

Which of the following are true of multiple-choice tests and questions?

A. The tests are very simplistic

B. The questions are easy to answer

C. The tests are a poor substitute for real examinations

D. A good guessing strategy will always get you a decent mark

E. None of the above

The answer, of course, is E – none of the above.

Multiple-choice tests have a very good track record in the field of assessment and, particularly, in selection. Multiple-choice questions are a technique that simply tests the candidates' knowledge and understanding of a particular subject on the date of the test. They make candidates read and think, but not write, about the question set, as is the case with essay-type questions.

It is true that there have been a number of long-held criticisms – and myths – about multiple-choice tests. For one, it has been a criticism that they are too simple-minded and trivial. What this observation really means is that it is perfectly obvious to the candidate what he or she has to do. There are no marks for working out what the examiner wants – it's obvious. But this is not the same as saying that the answer is obvious – far from it.

In addition, multiple-choice questions are often referred to by students as being 'multiple-guess' questions, on the basis that the right answer lies in one of the options given and therefore you have a good mathematical chance of happening upon the right answer. Although systematic and even completely random guessing does occur in multiple-choice tests, their effects can be minimised and their use identified by properly constructed, presented and timed tests. The people who design and analyse multiple-choice tests are often just as interested in what wrong answers you give as the right ones. This is because, apart from other things, patterns can be discerned and compared with others taking the same test, and tendencies towards certain answers (e.g. always choosing option B) will stand out.

In short, guessing is easy to spot and unlikely to succeed. Given that the purpose of the UKCAT is to inform the overall decision-making process in selecting you over your fellow applicants (rather than simply achieving a bad result or score), relying on guesswork is a poor strategy.

Multiple-choice tests are used extensively both in Europe and the USA, from staged tests in schools to university selection and assessment, to some of the most complex and high-stake professional trade qualifications. The strength of these tests is that they can provide fair and objective testing on a huge scale at small cost, in the sense that their administration is standardised and their developers can demonstrate that the results are not going to vary according to the marker – a criticism of essay-type tests. The format and design of the multiple-choice questions used for the UKCAT will undoubtedly follow the general educational model.

The following description of the format and design of multiple-choice questions has been informed by two publications. First, *Assessment and Testing: A Survey of Research* (University of Cambridge Local Examinations Syndicate, 1995). The University of Cambridge Local Examinations Syndicate has been in existence for over 130 years and prepares examinations for over 100 countries. Secondly, *Constructing Written Test Questions for the Basic Clinical Sciences* (second edition, Susan M. Case and David B. Swanson, National Board of Medical Examiners, 1998). The National Board of Medical Examiners, which is based in the USA, uses multiple-choice questions to test in excess of 100,000 medical students each year, including foreign doctors, at numerous sites throughout the world.

In all, multiple-choice testing – properly conducted – is well established, well respected and well used across the professional assessment world.

Multiple-choice questions: 'one best answer' format

There are a number of different formats that can be used for multiple-choice tests but the most common format is that taken from the 'one best answer' family. Generally this is the format used in the UKCAT subtests and is discussed in detail below in relation to each of the four subtests. However, before looking at the specific subtests it is useful first to understand the general structure of the 'one best answer' format.

The one best answer format is also known as 'A-type questions' and it is the most widely used format in multiple-choice tests. This format makes explicit the number of choices to be selected, and it usually consist of a *stem* and a *lead-in question*, followed by a series of *choices*, normally between three and five. To demonstrate this we will use a simple example taken from a typical numerical aptitude test.

Stem

The stem is usually a set of circumstances that can be presented in a number of different ways. The circumstances may be presented in a few simple sentences (as a document, a letter or some form of pictorial display) or may be presented in a longer passage (such as a newspaper article or an extract from a book or periodical). The stem provides all the information for the question that will follow.

A simple numerical aptitude stem could be:

A college had 20,000 students in 1999. Of these students, 8,000 studied a science subject.

Lead-in question

The lead-in question identifies the exact answer the examiner requires from the circumstances provided in the stem. For example, the lead-in question for the stem example given above would be:

What is the approximate ratio of students studying science to the total number of students at the college?

Choices

The choices provided will always consist of **one** correct answer. The remainder are incorrect answers, often referred to as 'distracters'.

For example, typical choices for the stem and lead-in question example given above could be:

A.   2:3

B.   2:5

C.   3:2

D.   3:5

Answer and rationale

Answer B is correct: 2:5.

Ratios: rule

A ratio allows one quantity to be compared with another quantity. Any two numbers can be compared by writing them alongside each other, with the numbers separated by a ratio sign (:).

The ratio of students studying science to the total number of students at the college?

Step 1: write the figures separated by the ratio sign with the number being compared first, so here 8,000:20,000.

Step 2: reduce these figure down if possible. Here they can be reduced to 8:20 by discounting the thousands and then further reduced by dividing both numbers by 4 to obtain 2:5.

Step 3: the ratio of students studying science compared with the total number of students at the college is 2:5.

Format of the Verbal Reasoning subtest

This subtest assesses your ability to think logically about written information and to arrive at a reasoned conclusion.

Stem

This stem will consist of reading passages usually taken from books, magazines, periodicals, pamphlets or newspapers.

Lead-in question

For each of the stems, there will be four separate lead-in statements. These statements will relate to the reading passage, and you will be required to determine whether the statement is true or false, or whether you cannot determine if the statement is true or false.

Choices

There will be three choices for each question: True, False or Can't Tell. Again, only **one** of these choices will be the correct answer and the remaining two choices will be incorrect.

Format of the Quantitative Reasoning subtest

This subtest assesses your ability to solve numerical problems. The format of the Quantitative Reasoning subtest is very similar to that described in the example above.

Stem

The stem will consist of tables, charts and/or graphs.

Lead-in question

For each of the stems (i.e. the tables, charts and/or graphs), there will be four separate lead-in questions.

Choices

There will be five choices for each question: A, B, C, D and E. Remember, there is only **one** correct answer and the remaining four choices will be incorrect.

Format of the Abstract Reasoning subtest

This subtest assesses your ability to infer relationships from information by convergent and divergent thinking.

Stem

The stem will consists of a pair of shapes known as 'Set A' and 'Set B'.

Lead-in question

For each pair of Set A and Set B shapes, there will be five 'Test Shapes' which represent five lead-in-questions.

Choices

For each of the five Test Shapes there will be three choices: Set A, Set B or Neither Set. Only **one** of the three choices is correct.

Format of the Decision Analysis subtest

This subtest assesses your ability to decipher and make sense of coded information and to make judgements which cannot be based on logical deduction alone.

Stem

In the stem you will be presented with one scenario and a significant amount of information together with terms that become progressively more complex and ambiguous.

Lead-in-questions

There will be 36 separate lead-in-questions based on the one scenario.

Choices

There will be either four or five choices for each question, A, B, C, D, and/or E. Whereas in the Quantitative Reasoning subtest only one answer is correct, in the Decision Analysis subtest there may be more than one answer that is correct. This should be clearly indicated in the lead-in-question.

How to approach multiple-choice questions

Whatever the purpose or the design of the test, it is worth bearing in mind some general rules to follow when answering multiple-choice questions. Clearly, your score should be higher if you attempt to answer all the questions in the test and avoid wild guessing. However, if you are running out of time you may attempt some 'educated' guesses but, where five options are available, this may prove difficult. If there are questions you are unsure of, you can place a mark against them for reviewing later.

Although it is often repeated at every level of testing and assessment in every walk of life, it is nevertheless worth reiterating – always read the questions carefully. It may help to read them more than once to avoid misreading a critical word(s). With the verbal reasoning and problem-solving tests in the UKCAT, careful reading of the words presented is crucial.

Where all the options, or some of the options, begin with the same word(s), or appear very similar, be sure to mark the correct option.

In relation to the Verbal Reasoning subtest, do not use your own knowledge or experience of the subject matter to influence your answers – even if your knowledge contradicts that of the author. The concept of this subtest is not to test individual prior knowledge – it is to present everyone competing against you with the same opportunity to demonstrate his or her skills and aptitudes. As such your answers should relate directly to:

■ your understanding of the passage you have read; and
■ the way in which the author has presented it to you, the reader.

Examine each passage to extract the main ideas and avoid making hasty conclusions.

The following four chapters contain details of the four UKCAT subtests and provide practice tests for each. By working through these chapters you will not only familiarise yourself with the format of these tests but will also speed up your reactions and give yourself the confidence to handle the differing style of questions involved successfully.

Format of the Non-Cognitive Analysis subtest

This subtest identifies the attributes and characteristics of robustness, empathy and integrity that contribute to successful health professional practice.

The format of this sub-test differs from the other four as there are no right or wrong answers. The questions will be statements presented in various formats which will require you to indicate how strongly you agree with each statement, how well it describes you or how true it is of you.

Chapter 8
The Verbal Reasoning subtest

This chapter will help you to:

▓ understand the purpose and the format of verbal reasoning tests

▓ prepare for the Verbal Reasoning subtest using general verbal-reasoning questions

▓ test your knowledge and understanding of verbal reasoning-type questions

▓ identify those verbal reasoning skills where development is required.

Introduction

Pearson VUE describes the purpose of this subtest as follows: 'The Verbal Reasoning subtest assesses a candidate's ability to read and think carefully about information presented in passages.'

In the commercial world, the Verbal Reasoning subtest described by Pearson VUE is a classic critical reasoning test. The notion that we all have 'thinking skills' or 'core skills' that should be transferable to all subject areas has attracted a great deal of academic interest. One of these 'core skills' is called 'critical thinking' and the vast number of books on the subject testifies to the interest in – and complexity of – the subject. Critical thinking is fundamentally concerned with the way arguments are structured and produced by whatever media: discussion, debate, a paper, a report, an article or an essay. The following are the generally accepted criteria for critical thinking:

▓ The ability to differentiate between facts and opinions.

▓ The ability to examine assumptions.

▓ Being open minded as you search for explanations, causes and solutions.

▓ Being aware of valid or invalid argument forms.

▓ Staying focused on the whole picture, while examining the specifics.

▓ Verifying sources.

▓ Deducing and judging inductions.

▓ Inducing and judging inductions.

- Making value judgements.
- Defining terms and judging definitions.
- Deciding on actions.
- Being objective.
- A willingness and ability always to look at alternatives.

The above is not meant to be an exhaustive list of all the criteria of critical thinking, but it provides an overview of some of the basic principles that underpin the Verbal Reasoning subtest.

When making selection decisions – whether they are for training, further education or for job appointments – the area of critical thinking/reasoning is deemed to be very important. This is largely because these skills are important in performing the roles themselves, particularly those in management. Graduate/managerial-level aptitude tests of verbal reasoning, which are basically assessing the understanding of words, grammar, spelling, word relationships, etc., may provide an objective assessment of a candidate's verbal ability.

However, these types of test are seen by some to lack face validity (that is, they do not appear to be job related) when used for graduate/managerial roles. People of this level often object to being given 'IQ tests' and prefer an assessment that appears to replicate, to some extent, the content of the job (i.e. critically evaluating reports). It is also believed by some that classic verbal reasoning tests do not provide an indication of an individual's ability to think critically. Therefore psychometrists have developed what are generally called critical reasoning tests, which are similar in format to the UKCAT and are described in the following section.

This chapter provides you with an opportunity to test your understanding and knowledge of the range of questions you are likely to be presented with in this UKCAT subtest. By taking this opportunity, you should be able to identify areas where you may need some development.

Verbal Reasoning subtest

The Verbal Reasoning subtest is an onscreen test that will consist of 44 items associated with 11 reading passages. Four statements will be presented with each passage and there are three answer options for each statement: True, False or Can't Tell. Each statement is presented with the passage on a separate screen with the three answer options below. A period of 22 minutes is allowed for the subtest, with one minute for administration time and the remaining 21 minutes to answer the questions.

Before attempting the practice questions based on the approach taken in the UKCAT, you should find it beneficial to work through the following questions. These passages and questions are formatted along the lines to be used in the UKCAT, using the response options of True, False or Can't Tell. The answers and the rationales for the correct answers follow each question.

The first passage is a relatively short paragraph followed by just one question. Subsequent passages will increase in size and the number of questions will increase to a maximum of four. The final passage, with its four questions, will serve as a 'trial run' prior to attempting the Verbal Reasoning practice subtest. This staged approach should develop your understanding of how this type of reasoning test is structured, and should also develop your confidence and ability when answering the questions.

Passages, response formats and example questions

The passages are normally extracts taken from various books, magazines, periodicals, pamphlets and newspapers. These passages are *not* a test of knowledge and may not include any medical or scientific-type matters. Each of the passages is intended to convey information or to persuade the reader of a point of view. You *must* assume that what is stated in each passage is factual and avoid drawing on your own knowledge or experience of any of the topics, which may contradict that of the author. Drawing on this assumption, read the passage carefully and decide whether the statement is True or False, or whether you Can't Tell without more information.

The definitions to be applied to each statement are as follows:

- *True*: this means that the statement is actually made in the passage, that it is implied or follows logically from the information in the passage.
- *False*: this means that the statement directly contradicts a statement made in, implied by or following logically from the passage.
- *Can't tell*: this means that there is insufficient information in the passage to arrive at a firm conclusion as to whether the statement is true or false.

Example questions

Example passage I: European Convention on Human Rights: Article 10 (Freedom of Expression)

Article 10(2) clearly allows for an individual's freedom of expression to be curtailed under a number of circumstances including the prevention of disorder or crime and the protection of morals. Balancing these competing needs is one area where the European Court of Human Rights has allowed a reasonable 'margin of appreciation'. Nevertheless, any restrictions on an individual's freedom of expression will be narrowly construed and closely scrutinised.

Demonstrators may be able to rely on Article 10 as a defence to a charge under the Public Order Act 1986 and hunt saboteurs bound over to keep the peace by magistrates have been able to show their rights have thereby been unjustifiably restricted.

Source: Blackstone's Police Manual. Volume 4. General Police Duties (Oxford University Press, 2006). © Fraser Sampson, 2006. By permission of Oxford University Press.

Example passage I: question 1

Hunt saboteurs who have invoked Article 10 of the Convention have been released from being bound over to keep the peace.

A. True

B. False

C. Can't Tell

Answer: False

In the final sentence of the passage, which relates to hunt saboteurs, it states that they will be released from being bound over where they have been able to show that their rights have been unjustifiable restricted. However, at the start of this sentence it clearly states 'may be able to rely on Article 10'. Therefore it is false to say that all hunt saboteurs will be so released from being bound over by invoking Article 10.

Example passage II: National Minimum Wage

National Minimum Wage (NMW) was 7 years old on 1 April 2006 and since its introduction in 1999 rates have continued to increase each year. When first introduced the minimum wage stood at £3.60 per hour whilst currently, for workers aged 22 and above, this has now risen to £5.05 per hour (£5.35 from 1 October 2006). The rate for workers aged 18–21 and those on a Government approved training scheme has also increased from £3.00 per hour in 1999 to £4.25 (£4.45 from 1 October 2006). And in addition a rate of £3.00 per hour was introduced on 1 October 2004 (£3.30 from 1 October 2006) for workers under 18 who are above compulsory school leaving age.

Source: HM Revenue and Customs Employer Bulletin, April 2006, Issue 23.

Example passage II: question 1

Workers aged 21 have not had as big an increase in the minimum wage over the past 7 years as those who are aged 22.

A. True

B. False

C. Can't Tell

Answer: True

In 1999 the minimum wage was £3.60 per hour and now, for workers aged 22, it has risen to £5.05 per hour, an increase of £1.45. For workers aged 18–21 it has risen from £3.00 per hour in 1999 to £4.25 per hour in 2006, an increase of £1.25. Therefore the increase in the minimum wage for those aged 22 and over is £0.20 more than those aged 18–21.

Example passage II: question 2

Since 1 October 1999 the rate for workers aged 16–18 has been £3.00 per hour.

A. True

B. False

C. Can't Tell

Answer: Can't Tell

The passage states that 'a rate of £3.00 per hour was introduced on 1 October 2004… for workers under 18 who are above compulsory school leaving age'. However, the passage does not provide what compulsory school leaving age is. Although you may personally know what this is, it is not stated in the passage and therefore you cannot determine the answer without further information.

Example passage III: withdrawal symptoms

The new health Bill, coming into force in summer 2007, provides that all enclosed public spaces and workplaces in England will be smoke-free. The Bill covers virtually all workplaces, including offices, manufacturing plants, schools, shops, restaurants and voluntary workplaces. Vehicles – as enclosed workplaces – will also be caught by the ban. The only exemptions will be workplaces where people also live, such as prisons, oil-rigs, residential care homes, and designated hotel bedrooms. But as in Scotland, the new no-smoking law for England won't say whether organisations should extend the ban to outdoor premises, erect smoking shelters, continue to allow customary smoking breaks, or outlaw smoking altogether. One of the keys to successfully implementing changes to smoking policies is consultation, which gives staff time to assimilate the reasons, benefits and timescales involved. Three months' consultation, followed by three months' notice of policy change would not be unusual, according to lawyers.

Source: 'Withdrawal Symptoms' (Penny Cottee, *People Management*, 4 May 2006). © People Management.

Example passage III: question 1

Staff working at hotels who 'live in' will not be subject to the same no-smoking requirements as the other guests in the hotel.

A. True

B. False

C. Can't Tell

Answer: True

One of the exemptions is workplaces where people also live, and this includes designated hotel bedrooms. However, it is logical to assume that staff bedrooms are separate within a hotel and therefore would not be subject to any 'smoke free' requirement. In any event, if staff were making use of hotel rooms these could be designated as 'smoking' if necessary.

Example passage III: question 2

The new health Bill requires that organisations provide three months' consultation before implementing the no-smoking policy.

A. True

B. False

C. Can't Tell

Answer: False

The passage does not state that it is a specific requirement of the Bill to provide three months' consultation. It is only according to lawyers and, one assumes, best practice that three months' consultation, followed by three months' notice of policy change, would not be unusual.

Example passage III: question 3

It will be the responsibility of organisations themselves to introduce and enforce the new no-smoking law in the workplace.

A. True

B. False

C. Can't Tell

Answer: Can't Tell

From the tenet of the passage it is logical to assume that the introduction of a smoke-free workplace will be the responsibility of individual organisations. However, it is not as clear cut in relation to the enforcement issue. The Bill may contain both a vicarious liability on the part of the organisation as well as a liability in relation to the individual 'breaking the law' (i.e. smoking in the workplace).

Example passage IV: enabling dyslexics to cope in employment

Sequencing difficulties affect the ability to plan and organise work and express ideas on paper and verbally. Inaccuracies may occur in word processing or writing typically involving letters, or words appearing the wrong order and words being left out or repeated. Written letters are often the mirror or reverse image of those they should have used, i.e. d for b, p for q, p for b, n for u, m for w. Rotation of numbers and letters through 180 degrees may occur, e.g. 6 to 9, b to q, p to d, n to u, and a to e. Curved characters may be reproduced as similar ones with straight strokes, e.g. u as v, 2 as z, s as 5, and 8 as B. Common tools to help with spelling, and grammar problems, such as dictionaries, thesauri and spell checkers can be difficult for dyslexics to use.

Source: 'Enabling dyslexics to cope in employment' (Patrick Packwood, *Selection and Development Review*, Volume 22, no. 1, 2006). © The British Psychological Society 2006.

Example passage IV: question 1
Dictionaries, thesauri and spell checkers do not help dyslexics with sequencing problems.

A. True

B. False

C. Can't Tell

Answer: False

The passage actually states that 'dictionaries, thesauri and spell checkers can be difficult for dyslexics to use'. It does not say that they do not help dyslexics with sequencing problems – therefore the answer is false.

Example passage IV: question 2
Common problems in relation to letters can be where dyslexics include the letter 'n', which, if written, could actually be an 'u' or even a 'v' dependent on their particular difficulties with sequencing.

A. True

B. False

C. Can't Tell

Answer: Can't Tell

In the passage it states that written letters are often the mirror or reverse image of those they should have used, and provides the example of 'n' to 'u'. The passage also discusses curved characters being reproduced as similar ones with straight strokes, and provides the example of 'u' to 'v. However, whether or not an 'n' could be reproduced as a 'v' is not discussed, but it may be that a dyslexic with image and curved character problems could write 'v' from an initial 'n'. More information would be required before a definitive true or false answer could be given.

Example passage IV: question 3
Considering written letters are often the mirror or reverse image of those they should have used, some people with dyslexia may write 'b' for 'd', or 'w' for 'm'.

A. True

B. False

C. Can't Tell

Answer: True

The letters 'b' for 'd' and 'w' for 'm' are still mirror or reverse images and, although these have not been used by the author in his examples, he does use 'd' to 'b' and 'm' to 'w' which can logically be transposed.

Example passage IV: question 4
Dyslexics with sequencing problems may find it difficult to provide a coherent structure when writing an essay or presenting a research paper.

A. True

B. False

C. Can't Tell

Answer: True

The passage specifically states that 'Sequencing difficulties affect the ability to plan and organise work and express ideas on paper and verbally'. It can be assumed, therefore, that dyslexics with sequencing problems would find difficulty in structuring an essay or presenting a research paper.

Verbal Reasoning practice subtest

For the purposes of this book, the Verbal Reasoning practice subtest provided below contains 30 items associated with eight reading passages, which is approximately two-thirds the length of the UKCAT subtest (44 items and 11 reading passages). These questions do not replicate those used in the UKCAT but are of the same format.

If the reader wants to simulate 'test conditions', he or she is advised to use rough paper to mark down his or her choice for each of the questions (i.e. True, False or Can't Tell). You should aim to complete the test within *15 minutes* (i.e. approximately two-thirds the time allowed for the actual subtest).

The correct answer and rationale to each of the questions are given in the section following the practice subtest.

Passage I: duties of charity trustees in respect of charity property

Money not needed for immediate expenditure should be invested. We recommend that if expenditure is expected in the near future, surplus cash is deposited to earn interest. Investments need to be reviewed periodically to ensure that they remain suitable for the charity's needs. Wherever possible, we suggest that funds are placed in a range of investments so as to avoid substantial losses caused by the failure of a single investment or institution. Bank accounts should be controlled by at least two of the trustees in the absence of explicit constitutional authority to do otherwise. It is unacceptable for either signatory to sign blank cheques for completion by the other signatory. Trustees need to ensure that property, which is permanent endowment, is preserved and invested in such a way as to produce funds for expenditure while at the same time safeguarding the real value of the invested funds.

Source: *Responsibilities of Charity Trustees* (Charity Commission for England and Wales, 2002).

Passage I: question 1
Where trustees find that investments are no longer suitable for the charity's needs, they must reinvest them, preferably in a range of other investments.

A. True

B. False

C. Can't Tell

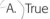

Passage I: question 2
The trustees may agree that the control of the bank accounts is undertaken by the treasurer (a trustee) and the chief executive of the charity (not a trustee).

A. True

B. False

C. Can't Tell

Passage I: question 3

The trustees must safeguard the real value of the invested funds, and any required expenditure should be obtained from surplus cash or investment funds from property.

A. True

B. False

C. Can't Tell

Passage I: question 4

Money needed for immediate expenditure would include the payment of staff salaries and other day-to-day expenditure of the charity.

A. True

B. False

C. Can't Tell

Passage II: aiming for excellence

For 2004–05, the Council has to report to the Audit Commission results against 56 Best Value Performance Indicators (BVPIs). In summary our performance against these indicators was: targets were set for 44 BVPIs and the Council reached or exceeded target for 35 BVPIs; 80 per cent of targets were reached or exceeded; 45 BVPIs were measured in both 2003–04 and 2004–05 and for these the Council's performance improved, or remained unchanged at the best performance possible; 62 per cent of indicators showed improvement or were unchanged at best possible performance; there are 34 BVPIs for which comparative data against all other similar councils is available and of these the Council achieved top-quartile performance against 18, i.e. for 53 per cent of our indicators the Council was among the top 25 per cent best performing councils in the country; we reached top-tier performance in 53 per cent of indicators.

Source: 'Aiming for excellence' (*South Shropshire Money Matters*, Spring 2006).

Passage II: question 5

In reality, the Council have only achieved top-quartile performance in just under a third of the Best Value Performance Indicators.

A. True

B. False

C. Can't Tell

Passage II: question 6

38 per cent of the 45 Best Value Performance Indicators measured in 2004–05 showed performance diminishing or a lack of improvement during this period.

A. True

B. False

C. Can't Tell

Passage II: question 7

53 per cent of the Council's Best Value Performance Indicators was among the top 25 per cent best performing councils in the country.

A. True

B. False

C. Can't Tell

Passage II: question 8

Of the Best Value Performance Indicators that were set by the Council for 2004–05, they only failed to reach or exceeded their target in relation to nine indicators.

A. True

B. False

C. Can't Tell

Passage III: degrees in two years

Students will be able to gain an honours degree in only two years as part of a 'study anytime' revolution for higher education.

Long summer holidays will end for undergraduates on 'compressed' degrees as they complete their studies a year early so that they can get on with their careers with reduced level of debt. Others will take courses entirely at work through online study in an effort to raise the proportion of adults with degree qualifications. They will be given credit towards their degrees for skills learnt on training courses.

A common system of American-style credit accumulation will also allow students to take study breaks and complete degrees later, possibly at different institutions.

Half of new British jobs will require a graduate qualification by 2012. While the numbers at university continue to rise the proportion of people entering higher education has stalled ·below 50 per cent – the Government target.

Source: 'Degrees in two years to ease student debt burden' (Tony Haplin, *The Times*, 18 April 2006). ©The Times.

Passage III: question 9

By reducing the length of 'holiday time' that undergraduates currently have, a three years' degree can be accomplished in two years.

A. True

B. False

C. Can't Tell

Passage III: question 10

Two-year degree programmes will mean that nationally students will have less debt when they leave than current undergraduates.

A. True

B. False

C. Can't Tell

Passage III: question 11

The Government considers that the current qualifications and skills of the adult working population are insufficient to meet the needs of the changing workplace.

A. True

B. False

C. Can't Tell

Passage III: question 12

The Government target is that 50 per cent of all new British jobs will be filled by graduates by 2012.

A. True

B. False

C. Can't Tell

Passage IV: International Standard Book Numbering (ISBN)

The purpose of the International Standard, is to co-ordinate and standardize the use of identifying numbers so that each international standard book number (ISBN) is unique to a title, or edition of a book, or other monographic publication published, or produced by a specific publisher or producer. It specifies the construction of an international standard book number and the location of the printed number on the publication.

This International Standard is applicable to books and other monographic publications, which may include: printed books and pamphlets (and their various bindings or formats), mixed media publications, other similar media including educational films/videos and transparencies, books on cassettes, microcomputer software, electronic publications, microfilms publications, Braille publications, and maps. Serial publications, music sound recordings and printed music are specifically excluded, as they are covered by other identification systems.

Source: *International Standard Book Numbering* (The Standard Book Numbering Agency Ltd, 2000).

Passage IV: question 13
The International Standard does not apply to written materials such as magazines, comics, short stories, holiday brochures, etc.

A. True

B. False

C. Can't Tell

Passage IV: question 14
A publisher does not need to obtain an ISBN for a new book that is about the development of computer websites where the book will only be accessible on the Internet and not in hard copy.

A. True

B. False

C. Can't Tell

Passage IV: question 15
In addition to its cataloguing properties, the International Standard also provides a policing function for new publications in ensuring that they are centrally registered and thereby eliminating non-standard practices and plagiarism.

A. True

B. False

C. Can't Tell

Passage IV: question 16

A local media company needs to obtain an ISBN for a video it has produced on behalf of the local district council to promote the local area for tourists and which will be sold at local outlets across the district.

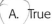
A. True

B. False

C. Can't Tell

Passage V: drug firms seek to stop generic HIV treatment

Until last year India permitted the copying of patented drugs, which allowed the country's pharmaceutical industry to sell cheap versions of Aids drug cocktails, known as antiretrovirals. Legislation enacted in March 2005 curtails the ability of firms to make copycat treatments and allow foreign pharmaceutical companies to claim ownership for drugs.

The Californian-based Gilead and Britain's GlaxoSmithKline, have now applied for patents on two HIV treatments. Campaigners, lawyers and Indian drug makers have opposed the applications, and more than 100 people were arrested in protests yesterday in Delhi.

Activists say patents would drive up prices as Indian manufacturers would have to pay royalties and rival generic versions would be blocked for 20 years.

Exports by Indian companies helped to cut the price of antiretroviral treatment from $15,000 (£8,000) per patient per year a decade ago to $200. Indian companies now provide two-thirds of the world's cheap Aids therapies.

Source: 'Drug firms seek to stop generic HIV treatment' (Randeep Ramesh, *Guardian*, 11 May 2006). ©The Guardian.

Passage V: question 17

The price of exports from India of antiretroviral treatment will rise by almost 100 per cent over the next decade to $15,000 per patient per year.

A. True

B. False

C. Can't Tell

Passage V: question 18

The reason the Indian Government has legislated to allow foreign pharmaceutical companies to claim ownership for drugs is to attract foreign drug companies, such as Gilead and GlaxoSmithKline, to bring further investment to the country.

A. True

B. False

C. Can't Tell

Passage V: question 19

Campaigners, lawyers and Indian drug makers are opposed to all applications for patents of HIV treatments from foreign pharmaceutical companies.

A. True

B. False

C. Can't Tell

Passage V: question 20

If Californian-based Gilead and Britain's GlaxoSmithKline are successful in their application for patents of HIV treatments in India, the cost of Aids therapies in two thirds of the world's markets will rise significantly.

A. True

B. False

C. Can't Tell

Passage VI: national debt

Government figures released yesterday showed that at the end of 2006, government net debt stood at £504.1bn, up from £467bn at the end of 2005. Public sector net borrowing – the government's preferred measure of its deficit – ran at £7.2bn last month which was enough to push overall debt above £500bn.

'Today's figures show that as each month passes Gordon Brown is losing control of the public finances. The Chancellor needs to stop dreaming about Number 10 and concentrate more on the economy,' said Vince Cable, the Liberal Democrat treasury spokesman.

As a percentage of the economy, however, the national debt is far lower than it has been in the past. It is currently 38.1 per cent of gross domestic product, lower than the 43.5 per cent that Labour inherited in 1997, but well up from the trough of 30.1 per cent seen in 2002 after the government had run budget surpluses for several years and had used £22bn of receipts from an auction of mobile phone spectrum to pay down debt.

Source: *National debt breaks through £500bn barrier* (Ashley Seager, *Guardian*, 20 January 2007). ©The Guardian.

Passage VI: question 21

Gordon Brown's dreams about Number 10 have contributed to his loss of control of the public finances.

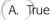
A. True

B. False

C. Can't Tell

Passage VI: question 22

Public sector net borrowing is the best measure of the level of national debt.

A. True

B. False

C. Can't Tell

Passage VI: question 23

As a percentage of the economy, the national debt is currently 8 per cent higher than the 10- year low but is 5.4 per cent lower than the 10-year high.

A. True

B. False

C. Can't Tell

Passage VI: question 24

The auction of mobile phone spectrum provided the largest revenue for the reduction of the 2002 national debt.

A. True

B. False

C. Can't Tell

Passage VII: China's satellite

The satellite occupied a region of space just over 500 miles high called low-Earth orbit. It is the lowest of the satellite orbits available and is favoured by the military for spy satellites, since it gives them the best possible images of the ground.

Despite picking off one of its lowest satellites in the test, China has developed two longer-range missiles, known as the KT-2 and KT-2A, which carry boosters and are believed to be capable of reaching more critical satellites in higher orbits.

The GPS satellites that are crucial for smart weapons, such as cruise missiles, orbit at about 8,000 miles above Earth, and broadband communications satellites orbit at around 22,000 miles in geostationary orbits. Together, GPS and communications satellites are Achilles' heels of modern warfare.

During the last Iraq war, 83 per cent of communications between allied forces were sent via satellites.

Source: Battering ram technology brought up to date for the 21st century (Ian Sample, *Guardian*, 20 January 2007). ©The Guardian.

Passage VII: question 25
China used one of its KT-2 range missiles to take out one of its low-Earth orbit satellites.

A. True

B. False

C. Can't Tell

Passage VII: question 26
Broadband satellites orbit the earth at almost three times the height of military satellites.

A. True

B. False

C. Can't Tell

Passage VII: question 27
Due to the vulnerability of satellites modern wartime communications are at greater risk than previous wartime methods of communication.

A. True

B. False

C. Can't Tell

Passage VII: question 28
High-orbit satellites cannot provide images of the ground.

A. True

B. False

C. Can't Tell

Passage VIII: a mountain on Crete

A blaze of wild flowers brightened the otherwise stark landscape as we set off up Crete's highest mountain. Psiloritis, 'the high one', better known as Mount Ida, is 2,456 metres high and often shrouded in cloud. But on this late spring day it had revealed its twin snow-capped peaks that tower over the central part of the island.

A good paved road winds its way up through the rocky slopes, past the round stone shepherd huts once used for watching summer flocks and making cheese and yoghurt. Griffon vultures circled overhead. We rounded a bend and suddenly found ourselves driving through low-lying clouds. This heavenly ascent was a fitting approach to the mountain's Idaean Cave, one of two caves on Crete vying for the title of the birthplace of Zeus.

Source: 'Land of myths and legends' (Donna Dailey, *RCI Holiday Magazine*, January 2007).

Passage VIII: question 29
There are two caves on the island of Crete.

A. True

B. False

C. Can't Tell

Passage VIII: question 30
Mount Psiloritis is to be found at the heart of the island of Crete.

A. True

B. False

C. Can't Tell

Verbal Reasoning practice subtest: answers

Question number	Correct response
1	B – False
2	C – Can't Tell
3	A – True
4	A – True
5	A – True
6	C – Can't Tell
7	B – False
8	A – True
9	A – True
10	C – Can't Tell
11	A – True
12	B – False
13	C – Can't Tell
14	A – False
15	B – False
16	C – Can't Tell
17	B – False
18	C – Can't Tell
19	A – True
20	C – Can't Tell
21	B – False
22	C – Can't Tell
23	A – True
24	C – Can't Tell
25	B – False
26	A – True
27	B – Can't Tell
28	B - False
29	C – Can't Tell
30	A – True

Verbal Reasoning practice subtest: explanation of answers

Passage I: duties of charity trustees in respect of charity property

Passage I: question 1

Where trustees find that investments are no longer suitable for the charity's needs, they must reinvest them, preferably in a range of other investments.

Answer: False

The passage states that investments need to be reviewed periodically to ensure that they remain suitable for the charity's needs and that, wherever possible, it is suggested, funds are placed in a range of investments. However, this is not categorical in that the investments must be placed in a range of investments. Therefore the answer is False.

Passage I: question 2

The trustees may agree that the control of the bank accounts is undertaken by the treasurer (a trustee) and the chief executive of the charity (not a trustee).

Answer: Can't Tell

In the passage it states that bank accounts should be controlled by at least two of the trustees in the absence of explicit constitutional authority to do otherwise. 'Explicit constitutional authority' is not expanded on, and it may be allowed for one trustee and another, in this instance the chief executive, to have control of the bank accounts or even other permutations. More information would be necessary and so the answer is Can't Tell.

Passage I: question 3

The trustees must safeguard the real value of the invested funds, and any required expenditure should be obtained from surplus cash or investment funds from property.

Answer: True

The answer is contained in the last sentence of the passage: 'Trustees need to ensure that property, which is permanent endowment, is preserved and invested in such a way as to produce funds for expenditure while at the same time safeguarding the real value of the invested funds.' Although property, which is permanent endowment, has been omitted from the question, it does not change the tenet of the passage and therefore the answer is True.

Passage I: question 4

Money needed for immediate expenditure would include the payment of staff salaries and other day-to-day expenditure of the charity.

Answer: True

In relation to money and expenditure, this is mentioned in the first two sentences of the passage: 'Money not needed for immediate expenditure should be invested. We recommend that if expenditure is expected in the near future, surplus cash is deposited to earn interest.' What constitutes 'immediate' is not really clear from the passage, though it might be assumed returns on investment money would have to be left within a fund for a considerable time to produce any return. It is logical to assume that staff salaries and day-to-day expenditure would constitute 'immediate expenditure' and therefore the answer is True.

Passage II: aiming for excellence

Passage II: question 5

In reality, the Council have only achieved top-quartile performance in just under a third of the Best Value Performance Indicators.

Answer: True

The first sentence of the passage states that there are 56 Best Value Performance Indicators. In the final sentence it states that the Council achieved top-quartile performance against 18 indicators. Because 18 as a fraction of 56 is just under a third, the answer is True.

Passage II: question 6

38 per cent of the 45 Best Value Performance Indicators measured in 2004–05 showed performance diminishing or a lack of improvement during this period.

Answer: Can't Tell

The passage states that 62 per cent of indicators showed improvement or were unchanged at best possible performance, which leaves 38 per cent of indicators unaccounted for in 2004–05. It might be assumed that performance against these indicators diminished or lacked improvement during this period. However, in relation to the 62 per cent of indicators, it is difficult to establish the precise meaning of the phrase 'best possible performance'. Does this phrase mean a 'lack of improvement' or was the rating already quite high at 'best possible performance'? It is impossible to determine without more information and so the answer is Can't Tell.

Passage II: question 7

53 per cent of the Council's Best Value Performance Indicators was among the top 25 per cent best performing councils in the country.

Answer: False

The figure '53 per cent' is mentioned twice in the final part of the passage: first, in relation to comparative achievement against other similar councils and, secondly, in stating that the Council reached top-tier performance in 53 per cent of indicators. The passage does not state that 53 per cent of its indicators were among the top 25 per cent best performing councils in the country and therefore the answer is False.

Passage II: question 8

Of the Best Value Performance Indicators that were set by the Council for 2004–05, they only failed to reach or exceeded their target in relation to nine indicators.

Answer: True

The passage may appear somewhat confusing in relation to the actual figures being used. At first it refers to setting 44 Best Value Performance Indicators and reaching or exceeding the target for 35 of these indicators. It then mentions measuring 45 indicators, with 62 per cent showing improvement or being unchanged at best possible performance. However, these latter measurement figures relate to both 2003–04 and 2004–05. It is the first set of figures that provides the answer (i.e. the 44 indicators of which 35 reached or exceeded the target in 2004–05). This would mean that the Council failed to reach or exceed its target in relation to nine indicators, and the answer to the question is True.

Passage III: degrees in two years

Passage III: question 9

By reducing the length of 'holiday time' that undergraduates currently have, a three years' degree can be accomplished in two years.

Answer: True

The passage actually states that 'Long summer holidays will end for undergraduates on "compressed" degrees as they complete their studies a year early'. It could be reasoned that there may be undergraduates who will not be on 'compressed' degrees. However, from the whole thrust of the passage it seems logical that full-time degree programmes of the future will be reduced to two years. There may also be other factors in relation to the reduced time, such as more lectures, tutorials, etc., but it can be assumed the reduction of 'holiday time' will be one of the major factors and therefore the answer to the question is True.

Passage III: question 10

Two-year degree programmes will mean that nationally students have less debt when they leave than current undergraduates.

Answer: Can't Tell

The passage states that, because students on two-year degree programmes will complete their studies early, they will have a reduced level of debt compared with current undergraduates. However, the statement refers to a reduction of the 'national' student debt. We are not told the actual figures of this debt. The two-year programmes may enable increased numbers to undertake degrees as undergraduates, thus raising the level of students nationally. The costs of tuition and other attendant costs may increase. These and other factors may mean an actual increase in the national student debt. So without more information the answer is Can't Tell.

Passage III: question 11

The Government considers that the current qualifications and skills of the adult working population are insufficient to meet the needs of the changing workplace.

Answer: True

Although this is not expressly stated it can be assumed from the information contained in the passage that the Government does consider that the adult working population needs an improvement in qualifications and skills. It intends enabling people to take courses entirely at work through online study in an effort to raise the proportion of adults with degree qualifications. In addition, the credit system envisaged will allow credit to be given for skills learnt on training courses, and the flexibility of the proposed system with study breaks, etc., can only assist adult learners. Therefore the answer is True.

Passage III: question 12

The Government target is that 50 per cent of all new British jobs will be filled by graduates by 2012.

Answer: False

The Government target mentioned in the passage relates to the number of people entering higher education and the fact that this has stalled at 50 per cent. In the same paragraph the passage also states that half of new British jobs will require graduate qualification by 2012. This is not indicated to be the Government target and so the answer is False.

Passage IV: International Standard Book Numbering (ISBN)

Passage IV: question 13

The International Standard does not apply to written materials such as magazines, comics, short stories, holiday brochures, etc.

Answer: Can't Tell

The passage states that the International Standard is applicable to books, etc., which may include books and pamphlets. There is no specific mention in the passage in relation to magazines, comics and holiday brochures. According to the passage, serial publications (e.g. comics and probably most magazines) do not need an ISBN. It could also be assumed that short stories are normally produced or published in the form of a book or pamphlet and therefore do need an ISBN. However, it is highly doubtful that holiday brochures would need an ISBN. With the exception of holiday brochures, it would also be necessary to obtain further information, in particular as to whether the 'serial publication' actually includes magazines and comics. On the basis of the holiday brochures alone, the answer to this question must be Can't Tell.

Passage IV: question 14

A publisher does not need to obtain an ISBN for a new book that is about the development of computer websites where the book will only be accessible on the Internet and not in hard copy.

Answer: False

The passage states that the International Standard is applicable to books and other monographic publications, which may include electronic publications. The production of the computer website book on the Internet would be an electronic publication and would require an ISBN, even if it is not produced in hard copy. Therefore the answer is False.

Passage IV: question 15

In addition to its cataloguing properties, the International Standard also provides a policing function for new publications in ensuring that they are centrally registered and thereby eliminating non-standard practices and plagiarism.

Answer: False

The passage states that the purpose of the International Standard is to co-ordinate and standardise the use of identifying numbers to ensure they are unique to the title or edition of the relevant publication. There is no suggestion, nor does it logically follow from the contents of the passage, that the standard has any type of policing role in eliminating non-standard practices and plagiarism, so the answer is False.

Passage IV: question 16

A local media company needs to obtain an ISBN for a video it has produced on behalf of the local district council to promote the local area for tourists and which will be sold at local outlets across the district.

Answer: Can't Tell

The only mention in the passage to videos relates to the requirement in relation to educational films/videos and transparencies. However, from the way the passage is worded (i.e. 'other similar media including'), the list provided is obviously not exhaustive and may well include videos other than those for an educational purpose. Therefore more information would be required, and so the answer is Can't Tell.

Passage V: drug firms seek to stop generic HIV treatment

Passage V: question 17

The price of exports from India of antiretroviral treatment will rise by almost 100 per cent over the next decade to $15,000 per patient per year.

Answer: False

The passage states that exports by Indian companies helped to cut the price of anti-retroviral treatment from $15,000 per patient per year a decade ago to $200. The question is suggesting that the reverse may occur if foreign pharmaceutical companies are allowed to claim ownership for drugs. This answer is therefore False as the passage does not present the information in this way.

Passage V: question 18

The reason the Indian Government has legislated to allow foreign pharmaceutical companies to claim ownership for drugs is to attract foreign drug companies, such as Gilead and GlaxoSmithKline, to bring further investment to the country.

Answer: Can't Tell

There is nothing in the passage to suggest that the Indian Government is trying to attract foreign investment by legislating to allow foreign pharmaceutical companies to claim ownership for drugs. It does sound a convincing reason and may even be the case, but more information would be required before this statement could be accepted. Therefore the answer is Can't Tell.

Passage V: question 19

Campaigners, lawyers and Indian drug makers are opposed to all applications for patents of HIV treatments from foreign pharmaceutical companies.

Answer: True

In the passage it states that campaigners, lawyers and Indian drug makers have opposed the applications for patents of HIV treatments from just two pharmaceutical companies, Gilead and GlaxoSmithKline. However, it is logical to assume that any similar applications for patents from foreign companies would be equally opposed, and therefore the answer is True.

Passage V: question 20
If Californian-based Gilead and Britain's GlaxoSmithKline are successful in their application for patents of HIV treatments in India, the cost of Aids therapies in two thirds of the world's markets will rise significantly.

Answer: Can't Tell

According to the passage, activists say patents would drive up prices as Indian manufacturers would have to pay royalties and rival generic versions would be blocked for 20 years. It also states that Indian companies now provide two thirds of the world's cheap Aids therapies. Although it appears likely that prices of treatments would rise in two thirds of the world's markets, whether or not this would be significant is not known. For instance, another country could take over from India to permit the copying of patented drugs, or the foreign drug companies could minimise the increase in costs or give concessions to third-world countries, etc. Therefore without more information the answer is Can't Tell.

Passage VI: national debt

Passage VI: question 21
Gordon Brown's dreams about Number 10 have contributed to his loss of control of the public finances.

Answer: False

The passage states that Gordon Brown is losing control of the public finances and that the Chancellor needs to stop dreaming about Number 10. Whilst this may or may not have some credence it is just the opinion quoted from Vince Cable, the Liberal Democrat treasury spokesman, and is more likely to be political sniping. Therefore, the answer is False.

Passage VI: question 22
Public sector net borrowing is the best measure of the level of national debt.

Answer: Can't Tell

The passage states that public sector net borrowing is the government's preferred measure of its deficit. It could be argued, therefore, that this is probably the best measure of the level of national debt but further information relating to other fiscal measures would be needed prior to making a decision. Therefore, the answer is Can't Tell.

Passage VI: question 23

As a percentage of the economy, the national debt is currently 8 per cent higher than the 10-year low but is 5.4 per cent lower than the 10-year high.

Answer: True

The passage gives the current percentage of 38.1 per cent and refers to the fact that Labour inherited a figure of 43.5 per cent in 1997, which is 10 years ago. It also states that a trough of 30.1 per cent was seen in 2002. Therefore the current 38.1 per cent is 8 per cent higher than the 10-year low of 30.1 per cent. In addition 38.1 per cent is 5.4 per cent lower than the 10-year high of 43.5 per cent which Labour inherited in 1997. Therefore, the answer is True.

Passage VI: question 24

The auction of mobile phone spectrum provided the largest revenue for the reduction of the 2002 national debt.

Answer: Can't Tell

The passage states that the government used £22bn of receipts from an auction of mobile phone spectrum to pay down debt. However, we are not provided with enough information regarding the actual level of reduction of debt in that year and the sources of revenue which made up the reduction. It is possible that the quoted amount was the largest contributor but we cannot tell this without further information. Therefore, the answer is Can't Tell.

Passage VII: China's satellite

Passage VII: question 25

China used one of its KT-2 range missiles to take out one of its low-Earth orbit satellites.

Answer: False

The passage states that despite picking off one of its lowest satellites, China has developed two longer-ranges missiles known as the KT-2 and KT-2A. Therefore, this implies that a previous version of missile was used to take out the low-Earth orbit satellite, prior to the development of the KT-2 range of missiles. Therefore, the answer is False.

Passage VII: question 26
Broadband satellites orbit the earth at almost three times the height of military satellites.

Answer: True

The passage states that satellites for smart weapons orbit above the earth at about 8,000 miles whilst communication satellites orbit at around 22,000 miles; 8,000 is approximately a third of 22,000, therefore broadband satellites orbit at almost three times the height of military satellites. Therefore, the answer is True.

Passage VII: question 27
Due to the vulnerability of satellites modern wartime communications are at greater risk than previous wartime methods of communication.

Answer: Can't Tell

The passage states that GPS and communications satellites are Achilles' heels of modern warfare and that during the last Iraq war 83 per cent of communication between allied forces was sent via satellites. It may be possible that other modern technological methods could still provide better methods of communication than previous wartime methods but this information is not available. Therefore, the answer is Can't Tell.

Passage VII: question 28
High-orbit satellites cannot provide images of the ground.

Answer: False

The passage states that a low-orbit satellite is favoured by the military for spy satellites, since it gives them the best possible images of the ground. It does not state that high-orbit satellites cannot provide images of the ground but it could be implied that the images would not have the same clarity. Therefore, the answer is False.

Passage VIII: a mountain on Crete

Passage VIII: question 29
There are two caves on the island of Crete.

Answer: Can't Tell

The passage states the mountain's Idaean Cave is one of two caves on Crete vying for the title of the birthplace of Zeus. It does not state that there are only two caves on the island of Crete, and although this may be true the information is not available in the passage. Therefore, the answer is Can't Tell.

Passage VIII: question 30

Mount Psiloritis is to be found at the heart of the island of Crete.

Answer: True

The passage states that Mount Psiloritis's, better known as Mount Ida's, twin snow-capped peaks tower over the central part of the island. Therefore, we could say that Mount Psiloritis is at the heart of the island of Crete. Therefore, the answer is True.

Chapter 9
The Quantitative Reasoning subtest

This chapter will help you to:

■ understand the purpose and the format of quantitative reasoning tests

■ prepare for the Quantitative Reasoning subtest using general numerical aptitude questions

■ test your knowledge and understanding of numerical-type questions

■ identify those numerical skills where development is required.

Introduction

Pearson VUE describes the purpose of this subtest as follows:

> The Quantitative Reasoning subtest assesses a candidate's ability to solve numerical problems. This subtest requires the candidate to solve problems by extracting relevant information from table and other numerical presentations. It assumes familiarity with numbers to a good pass at GCSE but the problems to be solved are less to do with numerical facility and more to do with problem solving (i.e. knowing what information to use and how to manipulate it using simple calculations and ratios). Hence it measures reasoning using numbers as a vehicle rather than measuring a facility with numbers.

As outlined in the Introduction to this part of the book, commercially produced numerical aptitude tests have been in existence for many years, mainly for use in the selection and assessment of staff. There have been numerous books written on how to pass or how to master psychometric tests, and what follows is a précis on what you need to consider specifically in approaching the Quantitative Reasoning subtest. Essentially, the advice on preparation for any aptitude test, contained in the first chapter, holds true for numerical tests.

Quite simply, numerical tests are designed to measure your ability to understand numbers. This relates to the four basic arithmetic operations of addition, subtraction, multiplication and division, as well as number sequences and simple mathematics. Therefore, in preparing for such tests, you need to be able to perform simple calculations without the use of a calculator.

This chapter provides you with an opportunity to test your understanding and knowledge of the range of questions you are likely to be presented with in the UKCAT. By taking this opportunity you should be able to identify any numerical areas which you may need to develop. Obviously, as with any other type of examination, numerical questions can be presented in a variety of ways. However, the basic computations used will always be the same. So learn or remind yourself of the basics. The section following the subtest provides the answers to the questions. This includes not only the correct answer and rationale but also the reasons why the other options are incorrect. In addition, this section also provides the 'mathematical rule' for each question. All this is designed to reinforce or build on your understanding and knowledge of the syllabus areas.

Quantitative Reasoning subtest

The subtest will consist of 40 items associated with 10 tables, charts and/or graphs, which means there will be four multiple-choice questions for each of the 10 tables, charts, etc. A period of 22 minutes is allowed for the test, with one minute for administration time and the remaining 21 minutes to answer the questions.

For the purposes of this chapter, a range of questions have been designed to cover relevant areas of the Level 2 and Level 3 Adult Numeracy Core Curriculum produced by the Qualifications Curriculum Authority. Level 3 is equivalent to GCSE standard, and a score of 21 or above (out of 30) on the practice test below equates to a Grade C or above at GCSE. This should be sufficient to deal with the scope of questions contained within the subtest. In reality, at this level, you should be getting all the questions correct.

The curriculum areas covered in the practice test are as follows:

- Basic arithmetic operations of addition, subtraction, multiplication and division.
- Powers and roots.
- Proportional change and ratios.
- Measurement of average and range to compare distributions, and estimate mean, median and range of grouped data.
- Conversion between fractions, decimals and percentages.
- Formulae, equations and expressions.
- Conversion of measurements between systems.

Response formats and example question

The type of format used in the Quantitative Reasoning subtest is the same as the one used as an example of multi-choice questions in the Introduction to this part of the book. That is, a *stem* in the form of a table, chart or graph, followed by a *lead-in question* and then five possible *choices* – A, B, C, D or E.

Example question

The following example requires you to select the correct answer from the five options provided. The rationale for the correct and incorrect answers is provided after the question.

The table below shows the miles travelled by a sales representative.

	Mon	Tue	Wed	Thu	Fri	Sat
WEEK 1	197.5	189	213.5	231	190	437
WEEK 2	116.5	145	202	173	52	

You want to find her median mileage over the 11 days. Which of these would you do?

A.   Find the sixth number and divide this by 2

B.   Add all the numbers together and divide by 11

C.   Rearrange the numbers into numerical order and then find the sixth number

D.   Find the average for each week and divide this by 2

E.   Add the two middle numbers together and divide this by 2

Median: rule
The median of a distribution is the middle value when the values are arranged in order. When there are two middle values (i.e. for an even number of values), you add the two middle numbers and divide by 2.

Answer C is correct: Rearrange the numbers into numerical order and then find the sixth number.

Rationale
There are 11 values, an odd number, so arrange the values into numerical order and then find the middle value, which is the sixth number, and this is the median.

A is incorrect: Find the sixth number and divide this by 2. Here there is an odd amount of values so there is no need to divide anything by 2, only find the middle value.

B is incorrect: Add all the numbers together and divide by 11. This is the method for finding the mean, not the median.

D is incorrect: Find the average for each week and divide this by 2. This is not a method for finding any type of average.

E is incorrect: Add the two middle numbers together and divide this by 2. This is the method of finding the median when there are an even number of values.

Quantitative Reasoning practice subtest

The practice test provided below contains 30 items with eight tables, charts and/or graphs. This represents the format of the Quantitative Reasoning subtest, though it only includes three-quarters the quantity of items. These questions do not replicate those used in the UKCAT but are of the same format.

If you want to simulate 'test conditions', you are advised to use rough paper to mark down your choice for each of the questions (i.e. A, B, C, D or E). You should aim to complete the test within *17 minutes* (i.e. three-quarters the time allowed for the subtest). The answers can then be checked against the 'answers' in the following section. Obviously, incorrect answers may identify a development need in a particular area of the syllabus. The rough paper can also be used for making any calculations. In the UKCAT, rough paper will not be available. There will be a portable whiteboard and pen for your personal use during the test.

Remember that each of the questions is always accompanied by five possible answers (A, B, C, D and E), and that only **one** answer is correct.

Also remember to read through all five competing answers before selecting what you consider to be the correct answer. By reading the four 'incorrect' answers you should confirm that your choice is in fact correct.

Questions 1 to 4 are based on the information in the tables below:

Findaphone: Pay As U Call

Cost of phone	£49.99		
Cost of calls per minute	£5 voucher	£10 voucher	£50 voucher
Peak rate	40p	35p	25p
Off-peak rate	10p	5p	2p

Lemon monthly 400

Cost of phone	Free
Connection fee	Free
Monthly line rental *(including 400 free off-peak minutes)	£15*
Cost of calls per minute: Peak rate Off-peak rate	 25p 1p

1   Bryony wishes to buy a mobile phone and has narrowed it down to the two possibilities shown above. She estimates that she will use 5 minutes peak rate and 10 minutes off-peak rate in phone calls per day.

How much will it cost Bryony in calls using Findaphone for one month (30 days), ignoring the cost of the phone, if she buys £10 vouchers?

A.   £43.50

B.   £52.50

C.   £67.50

D.   £72.50

E.   £90.00

2   If Bryony uses Findaphone for one month (30 days) with £5 vouchers, ignoring the cost of the phone, approximately how much more, expressed as a percentage, would this cost than using £10 vouchers?

A.   25%

B.   33%

C.   34%

D.   68%

E.   75%

3   Bryony chooses a 'Lemon' phone and keeps a record of the minutes she uses for 1 year. From this she draws the following chart:

Month	Peak rate	Off-peak rate
January	42	127
February	68	109
March	33	76
April	52	134
May	45	85
June	84	114
July	77	125
August	49	108
September	46	94
October	53	146
November	47	84
December	88	136

Her phone company, Lemon, tells Bryony that, as part of a promotion, she can claim back the mean average of her off-peak calls for one year and 50 per cent of the mean average of her peak calls for one year.

How many minutes can Bryony claim back to the nearest minute?

A.   57

B.   111.5

C.   112.75

D.   140

E.   168.5

4 As an alternative promotion, Bryony can choose to have her mobile phone upgraded.

	Current phone	Upgraded phone
Standby time	55 hours	72 hours
Talk time	⅓ of standby time	¼ of standby time
Charge time	1/20 of standby time	1/30 of standby time

Which of the following statements is true?

A. The current phone has longer talk time and longer charge time

B. The upgraded phone has longer talk time and longer charge time

C. The current phone has longer talk time and shorter charge time

D. The upgraded phone is quickest to charge and has the shortest standby time

E. The current phone has shorter talk time and longer charge time

Questions 5 to 8 are about the following table that shows a list of videos and their running times, in minutes:

Disney films	Running time	Other films	Running time
Flubber	90	Chitty Chitty Bang Bang	144
Toy Story	77	South Park	78
A Bug's Life	93	The Mask	97
Hercules	89	Small Soldiers	106
Lady and the Tramp	73	The Lost World	123
The Aristocats	77	The Rugrats Movie	77
Bambi	67	James and the Giant Peach	76
Cinderella	70	Men in Black	94
Peter Pan	74	Mouse Hunt	94
Lion King	84	Star Wars I – The Phantom Menace	127

5 What is the mean running time of the Disney films?

   A. 10

   B. 79.4

   C. 93

   D. 158.8

   E. 794

6 What is the median running time of the 'Other' films?

   A. 77

   B. 94

   C. 95.5

   D. 97

   E. 101.6

7 What can you say about the range of running times of the Disney films compared with the range of running times of the 'Other' films?

   A. The mode for the 'Other' films is lower

   B. It is longer

   C. They are the same

   D. The median for the Disney films is higher

   E. It is shorter

8 What is the mode running time of the Disney films?

   A. 74

   B. 76.5

   C. 77

   D. 90

   E. 94

Questions 9 to 12 refer to the pie chart below, which groups the level of turnover of a number of organisations included in a business sector survey. The number of organisations per group is shown in parentheses.

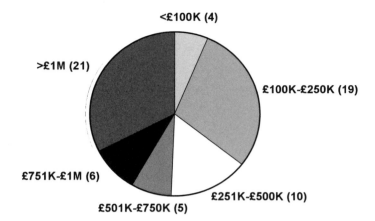

9   What percentage, to two decimal places, of organisations has a turnover in excess of £1M?

   A.   49.53%

   B.   46.34%

   C.   32.31%

   D.   57.89%

   E.   62.16%

10   What is the ratio of the number of organisations with a turnover of £501K–£750K compared with the rest of the organisations?

   A.   1:5

   B.   4:9

   C.   1:10

   D.   1:12

   E.   1:15

11   The Learning and Skills Council have asked the publishers of this business sector information also to produce the turnover of the organisations in euros. In converting pounds sterling to euros, where £1 = €1.45, what would be the minimum range figure in euros for those organisations with a turnover of £251K–£500K?

   A.   €145,000

   B.   €362,500

   C.   €363,950

   D.   €725,000

   E.   €726,450

12 The 65 organisations in this survey employ a total of 850 people of which about 63 per cent are employed by those organisations with a turnover in excess of £1M. The remaining employees are spread pro rata across the other organisations. How many employees, to the nearest round number, work for a company with a turnover of £251K–£500K?

A. 7

B. 12

C. 15

D. 19

E. 26

Questions 13 to 16 are about the table below, which shows the heights of 45 shop buildings measured to the nearest 0.1 metres.

Height in metres	2–2.9	3–3.9	4–4.9	5–5.9	6–6.9	7–7.9
Number of shop buildings	3	6	12	15	7	2

13 How many shop buildings are less than 5 metres high?

A. 6

B. 9

C. 12

D. 15

E. 21

14 What can you say that 20 per cent of the shop buildings are?

A. At least 5 metres high

B. At least 3 metres and less than 6 metres high

C. Less than 4 metres high

D. Less than 5 metres high

E. At least 7 metres high

15 What fraction of the shop buildings are between 5 and 5.9 metres high?

A. ⅓

B. ½

C. ¼

D. ⅜

E. ¾

16 Ten years after this data was collected, a further survey found that there had been the following increases, shown in parenthesis, in the number of shop buildings at the heights indicated: 3–3.9 (4); 4–4.9 (7); 5–5.9 (5); 6–6.9 (7); 7–7.9 (4). In calculating the revised total number of shop buildings and heights, what is the ratio of the shop buildings that are less than 5 metres compared with those that are 5 metres and above?

A. 3:4

B. 4:5

C. 5:6

D. 5:8

E. 7:10

Questions 17 to 20 are about the following table, which shows various types of biscuits sold by a national supermarket chain with their fat content in grams per 100 g.

Digestive	4.2	Shortbread	4.5
Jammy Dodgers	3.0	Morning Coffee	2.0
Custard Creams	0.9	Hobnobs	5.0
Bourbons	1.0	Ginger Nuts	2.0
Chocolate Digestive	4.5	Oat Crunch	3.9
Figs	1.0	Chocolate Fingers	2.6
Malted Milk	2.1	Jaffa Cakes	0.9
Nice	2.0	Honey Nuts	4.2
Rich Tea	3.0	Arrow Root	2.1
Garibaldi	1.0		

Sharon designs the table below to show the numbers of brands in five categories.

Amount of fat	Number of brands
Very low fat (0–1 g)	5
Low fat (1.1–2 g)	3
Medium fat (2.1–3 g)	5
High fat (3.1–4 g)	1
Very high fat (4.1–5 g)	4

Sharon then checks her table.

17 Is there anything wrong with the total number of brands in her table?

A. One too few

B. Two too few

C. One too many

D. Two too many

E. Total number of brands correct

18 One packet of digestives weighs 150 g and one packet of shortbreads weighs 130 g. If you bought 5 packets of digestives and 5 packets of shortbreads, what would be the difference in the fat content between the two types?

A. 0.3 g

B. 1.5 g

C. 1.75 g

D. 2.05 g

E. 2.25 g

19 Sharon is asked to find the median fat content of all the types of biscuits. Which of the following would she do?

A. Find the tenth number and divide this by 2

B. Add all the numbers together and divide by 19

C. Find the average and divide by 2

D. Rearrange the numbers into numerical order and then find the tenth number

E. Find the fat content figure that occurs most frequently

20 Sharon receives a request for the fat content of 25 100-gram packets of digestives to be provided in ounces. Grams (G) are converted to ounces (X) by dividing grams (G) by 28.3. Which option is the correct formula?

A. $X = 25 \dfrac{G}{(28.3)}$

B. $G = \dfrac{25X}{(28.3)}$

C. $G = \dfrac{25}{28.3X}$

D. $X = 28.3 \dfrac{G}{(25)}$

E. $X = \dfrac{28.3}{(25G)}$

Questions 21 to 23 are about a lunchtime menu at a motorway services.

21 At the motorway services the self-service restaurant shows the following hot meals available at lunchtime.

HOT FOOD LUNCH-TIME	
Sausage and Mash	£3.20
Fish and Chips	£3.50
Curry and Rice	£3.80
All Day Breakfast	£4.45
Vegetarian Pancake	£3.00
Chips – per portion	£1.20
Coffee	£0.75

You order one sausage and mash, one fish and chips and one vegetarian pancake with a portion of chips.

What is the total cost of the food you have ordered?

A. £7.90

B. £9.70

C. £10.90

D. £12.10

E. £7.40

22 The following day you order an All Day Breakfast and a coffee.

If you paid with a £10 note, how much change would you get?

A. £4.50

B. £4.80

C. £5.80

D. £6.20

E. £5.20

23 If you ignore the cost of a portion of chips and coffee, what is the range of the prices of the food?

A. 95p

B. £1.00

C. £1.45

D. £1.55

E. £3.00

Questions 24 to 26 relate to the following chart that shows the weights in kg of 25 fish caught by Bob the angler.

2.2	2.9	4.3	2.9	3.4
2.0	2.3	2.9	3.3	5.3
1.9	1.8	2.3	2.6	1.9
5.6	2.7	2.8	2.8	2.9
2.5	1.7	2.8	1.9	2.5

24 Any fish weighing 1.9 kg or less, Bob threw back into the river.

What percentage of fish did Bob throw back into the river?

A. 16%

B. 32%

C. 40%

D. 60%

E. 20%

25 What would be the proportion of fish, expressed as a fraction, that Bob threw back into the river if the weight had been 2.9 kg instead of 1.9 kg?

A. $\frac{1}{2}$

B. $\frac{2}{3}$

C. $\frac{3}{4}$

D. $\frac{4}{5}$

E. $\frac{1}{3}$

26 What is the ratio of the number of fish that Bob threw back into the river compared with the number of fish he did not?

A. 1:4

B. 1:3

C. 2:5

D. 2:3

E. 1:5

Questions 27 to 30 are about the chart below which shows the life span, in hours, for 20 Mini-Disc player batteries.

27 What is the percentage of batteries lasting less than 4 hours?

Battery no.	Life span	Battery no.	Life span
1	9	11	4
2	8	12	4
3	7	13	4
4	7	14	3
5	6	15	3
6	6	16	3
7	6	17	3
8	5	18	2
9	5	19	2
10	5	20	1

A. 25%

B. 35%

C. 55%

D. 65%

E. 20%

28 What is the mode of the batteries' life span?

A. 3

B. 4

C. 4.5

D. 6

E. 5

29 What is the range of the batteries' life span?

    A. 1

    B. 8

    C. 9

    D. 20

    E. 10

30 What is the mean of the batteries' life span?

    A. 3

    B. 8

    C. 4.5

    D. 9

    E. 4.65

Quantitative Reasoning practice subtest: answers

Question number	Correct response
1	C
2	B
3	D
4	A
5	B
6	C
7	E
8	C
9	C
10	D
11	C
12	A
13	E
14	C
15	A
16	B
17	A
18	E
19	D
20	A
21	C
22	B
23	C
24	E
25	D
26	A
27	B
28	A
29	B
30	E

Quantitative Reasoning practice subtest: explanation of answers

Question 1

Multi-stage calculations: rule
This question contains multiplication and addition.

Answer C is correct: £67.50.

Rationale
Step 1: gather all the relevant information required for the calculations. Findaphone: 30 days' use; £10 voucher which charges 35p peak rate and 5p off-peak; Bryony uses, per day, 5 minutes peak rate and 10 minutes off-peak.

Step 2: calculate the cost used per day so peak rate is $5 \times 35p = £1.75$ and off-peak is $10 \times 5p = 50p$.

Step 3: therefore the cost per month (30 days) is $(£1.75 + £0.50) \times 30 = £67.50$.

Answer A is incorrect: £43.50. Using approximations we can round the cost per day from £2.25 to £2 per day, then the cost per month (30 days) would be $£2 \times 30 = £60$. We know that because we rounded down in our approximations that the actual cost must be greater than £60 – therefore this option is incorrect.

Answer B is incorrect: £52.50. You would have to do the full calculations to disregard this option.

Answer D is incorrect: £72.50. You would have to do the full calculations to disregard this option.

Answer E is incorrect: £90.00. Using approximations we can round the cost per day from £2.25 to £3 per day, then the cost per month (30 days) would be $£3 \times 30 = £90$. We know that because we rounded up in our approximations that the actual cost must be less than £90 – therefore this option is incorrect.

Question 2

Percentage change: rule
To work out the **percentage change**, work out the increase or decrease and add or subtract it from the original amount. Percentage change = (Change ÷ Original amount) $\times$ 100%, where the change might be an increase, decrease, profit, loss, error, etc.

Answer B is correct: 33%.

Rationale

Step 1: gather all the relevant information required for the calculations. Findaphone: 30 days' use; £5 voucher which charges 40p peak rate and 10p off-peak; Bryony uses, per day, 5 minutes peak rate and 10 minutes off-peak.

Step 2: calculate the cost used per day, so peak rate is 5 × 40p = £2 and off-peak is 10 × 10p = £1.

Step 3: therefore the cost per month (30 days) is (£2 + £1) × 30 = £90.

Step 4: increase = £90 – £67.50 = £22.50.

Step 5: Percentage increase = (Increase ÷ Original amount) × 100% = $\frac{22.5}{67.50}$ × 100% = 33.33% (to 2 decimal places) = 33% (to the nearest whole number).

Answer A is incorrect: 25%. You would have to do the full calculations to disregard this option.

Answer C is incorrect: 34%. You would have to do the full calculations to disregard this option.

Answer D is incorrect: 68%. A 68% increase on £67.50 would be much higher than £22.50 and so this option can be disregarded.

Answer E is incorrect: 75%. A 75% increase on £67.50 would again be much higher than £22.50 and so this option can be disregarded.

Question 3

Mean: rule

The **mean** (or arithmetic mean) of a distribution is found by summing the values of the distribution and dividing by the number of values.

Answer D is correct: 140.

Rationale

Step 1: the mean of off-peak calls is the sum of the values divided by the number of values. Therefore 1338/12 = 111.5.

Step 2: the mean of peak calls is the sum of the values divided by the number of values. Therefore 684/12 = 57.

Step 3: 50% of the mean of peak calls is half of 57, so it is 28.5.

Step 4: in total, Bryony can claim 111.5 + 28.5 = 140 minutes.

Answer A is incorrect: 57. This is the mean of the peak calls. This value needs to be halved and then added to the mean of the peak calls.

Answer B is incorrect: 111.5. This is the mean of the off-peak calls. This value needs to be added to 50% of the mean of the peak calls.

Answer C is incorrect: 112.75. This is 50% of the mean of the off-peak calls added to the mean of the peak calls. It should have been 50% of the mean of the peak calls added to the peak calls.

Answer E is incorrect: 168.5. This is the mean of the off-peak calls, 111.5 plus the mean of the peak calls, 57, which equals 168.5. This option is incorrect as it is only 50% of the mean of the peak calls that is required.

Question 4

Fractions: rule
To find the **fraction** of an amount you must first divide the amount by the denominator (the number on the bottom) and multiply by the numerator (the number on the top).

Answer A is correct. The current phone has longer talk time and longer charge time.

Rationale
Step 1: for the current phone the standby time is 55 hours. The talk time is therefore one third of the standby time, so $55 \div 3 = 18.33$ hours (to 2 decimal places) and the charge time is one twentieth of the standby time, so $55 \div 20 = 2.75$ hours.

Step 2: for the upgraded phone the standby time is 72 hours. The talk time is therefore one quarter of the standby time, so $72 \div 4 = 18$ hours and the charge time is one thirtieth of the standby time, so $72 \div 30 = 2.4$ hours.

Step 3: the current phone has longer talk time and longer charge time.

Answer B is incorrect: The upgraded phone has longer talk time and longer charge time. The upgraded phone has 18 hours talk time and the current phone has 18.33 hours talk time – therefore this statement is incorrect.

Answer C is incorrect: The current phone has longer talk time and shorter charge time. The current phone has 2.75 hours charge time and the upgraded phone has 2.4 hours charge time – therefore this statement is incorrect.

Answer D is incorrect: The upgraded phone is quickest to charge and has the shortest standby time. The current phone has 55 hours standby time and the upgraded phone has 72 hours standby time – therefore this statement is incorrect.

Answer E is incorrect: The current phone has shorter talk time and longer charge time. The current phone has longer talk time (18.33 hours as opposed to 18 hours for the upgraded phone) – therefore this statement is incorrect.

Question 5

Mean: rule

The **mean** (or arithmetic mean) of a distribution is found by summing the values of the distribution and dividing by the number of values.

Answer B is correct: 79.4.

Rationale

Step 1: Mean = Sum of values ÷ Number of values.

Step 2: $\dfrac{90 + 77 + 93 + 89 + 73 + 77 + 67 + 70 + 74 + 84}{10}$

Step 3: Mean = 794 ÷ 10 = 79.4 minutes.

Answer A is incorrect: 10. This is the number of values in the distribution of Disney films and not the mean.

Answer C is incorrect: 93. This is the extreme upper value of the Disney films (i.e. the longest running time of the Disney films) and not the mean.

Answer D is incorrect: 158.8. This is the sum of the value (794) divided by half the number of values (5), whereas the number of values is actually 10.

Answer E is incorrect: 794. This is the sum of the values; it needs to be divided by the number of values, which is 10, to find the mean.

Question 6

Median: rule

The **median** of a distribution is the middle value when the values are arranged in order. When there are two middle values (i.e. for an even number of values), you add the two numbers and divide by 2.

Answer C is correct: 95.5.

Rationale

Step 1: arrange the values in order – so 76, 77, 78, 94, 94, 97, 106, 123, 127, 144.

Step 2: there is an even amount of values, so the median is $\dfrac{94 + 97}{2}$ = 95.5 minutes, as 94 and 97 are the 'middle' values in the distribution.

Answer A is incorrect: 77. This is the middle value, the median running time, of the Disney films.

Answer B is incorrect: 94. This is the 5th value in the distribution and not the middle value; the median is halfway between 94 and 97.

Answer D is incorrect: 97. This is the 6th value in the distribution and not the middle value; the median is halfway between 94 and 97.

Answer E is incorrect: 101.6. This is the mean of the 'Other' films and not the median.

Question 7

Range: rule
The **range** of a distribution is found by working out the difference between the highest value and the lowest value. The range should always be given as a single value.

Answer E is correct: It is shorter.

Rationale
Step 1: Disney films greatest value = 93. Lowest value = 67. The range = Greatest value – Lowest value = 93 – 67 = 26 minutes.

Step 2: 'Other' films greatest value = 144. Lowest value = 76. The range = Greatest value – Lowest value = 144 – 76 = 68 minutes.

Step 3: therefore the range of the Disney films is shorter than that of 'Other' films.

Answer A is incorrect: The mode for the 'Other' films is lower. This answer is incorrect as the mode is irrelevant to calculating the range.

Answer B is incorrect: It is longer. The range of 'Other' films is greater than the range of Disney films. Therefore this option is incorrect.

Answer C is incorrect: They are the same. The range of the 'Other' films is 68 and the range of Disney films is 26. Therefore the ranges are not the same.

Answer D is incorrect: The median for the Disney films is higher. This answer is incorrect as the median is irrelevant to calculating the range.

Question 8

Mode: rule
The **mode** is the number in a distribution that has the highest frequency – that is, it appears the most times in a collection of values.

Answer C is correct: 77.

Rationale
The value 77 appears the most times (twice) in the list of Disney films.

Answer A is incorrect: 74. This value appears in the list of Disney films but it does not appear more times than any other value so it is not the mode.

Answer B is incorrect: 76.5. This value does not appear at all in the list of running times for the Disney films.

Answer D is incorrect: 90. This value appears in the list of Disney films but it does not appear more times than any other value so it is not the mode.

Answer E is incorrect: 94. This is the mode running time of the 'Other' films.

Question 9

Percentages: rule
To express one number as a **percentage** of another, write the first number as a fraction of the second and convert the fraction to a percentage by multiplying it by 100.

Answer C is correct: 32.31%.

Rationale
Step 1: the number of organisations with a turnover in excess of £1M = 21. The number of organisations in the sample = 65.

Step 2: 21 as a fraction of the 65 = $\frac{21}{65}$.

Step 3: convert to a percentage, so $\frac{21}{65} \times 100 = 32.31\%$.

Step 4: therefore 32.31% of the organisations have a turnover in excess of £1M.

Answer A is incorrect: 49.53%. Using approximations, we know that 50 per cent of something is half of it and a half of 65 is approximately 33, so this cannot be the correct answer as we know the number of organisations with a turnover in excess of £1M is 21 and therefore a percentage figure considerably less than 50 per cent.

Answer B is incorrect: 46.34%. Using approximations, we know that 50 per cent of something is half of it and a half of 65 is approximately 33, so this cannot be the correct answer as the number of organisations with a turnover in excess of £1M is 21 and therefore a percentage figure less than 50 per cent. However, this option would have to be calculated to ensure the answer was incorrect.

Answer D is incorrect: 57.89%. Using approximations, we know that 50 per cent of something is half of it and a half of 65 is approximately 33. There are 21 organisations with a turnover in excess of £1M, so the answer must be under 50 per cent.

Answer E is incorrect: 62.16%. Using approximations, we know that 50 per cent of something is half of it and a half of 65 is approximately 33, so this cannot be the correct answer as the number of organisations with a turnover in excess of £1M is 21 and therefore a percentage considerably under 50 per cent.

Question 10

Ratios: rule
A **ratio** allows one quantity to be compared with another quantity. Any two numbers can be compared by writing them alongside each other with the numbers separated by a ratio sign (:).

Answer D is correct: 1:12.

Rationale
Step 1: five organisations have a turnover of £501K–£750K and therefore 65 – 5 = 60 organisations have a different turnover.

Step 2: write the figures separated by the ratio sign with the number being compared first, so here 5:60.

Step 3: reduce these figures down if possible. Both can be divided by 5 to give 1:12.

Step 4: the ratio of the number of organisations with a turnover of £501K–£750K compared with the rest of the organisations is 1:12.

Answer A is incorrect: 1:5. Multiplying both sides of this ratio by 5 gives 5:25 and so this option cannot be correct, as the ratio is 5:60.

Answer B is incorrect: 4:9. Multiplying both sides of this ratio by 5 gives 20:45 and so this option cannot be correct, as the ratio is 5:60.

Answer C is incorrect: 1:10. Multiplying both sides of this ratio by 5 gives 5:50 and so this option cannot be correct, as the ratio is 5:60.

Answer E is incorrect: 1:15. Multiplying both sides of this ratio by 5 gives 5:75 and so this option cannot be correct, as the ratio is 5:60.

Question 11

Conversion: rule
The equation for **converting** pounds to euros is $€ = £ \times 1.45$.

Answer C is correct: €363,950.

Rationale
Step 1: $€ = £ \times 1.45$.

Step 2: substitute £ with 251,000, so $€ = 251{,}000 \times 1.45$.

Step 3: $€ = 363{,}950$.

Answer A is incorrect: €145,000. This conversion is from £100K (i.e. € = 100,000 × 1.45 = €145,000).

Answer B is incorrect: €362,500. This conversion is from £250K (i.e. € = 250,000 × 1.45 = €362,500).

Answer D is incorrect: €725,000. This conversion is from £500K (i.e. € = 500,000 × 1.45 = €725,000).

Answer E is incorrect: €726,450. This conversion is from £501K (i.e. € = 501,000 × 1.45 = €726,450).

Question 12

Percentage and proportion: rule

To find the **percentage** of an amount, find 1% of the amount and then multiply to get the required amount. This question also contains subtraction and division.

Answer A is correct: 7.

Rationale

Step 1: find 1% of the amount (850 ÷ 100 = 8.5).

Step 2: multiply by the percentage required (8.5 × 63 = 535.5).

Step 3: find the remaining number of employees (850 − 535.5 = 314.5).

Step 4: divide the remaining employees by the number of other organisations (314.5 ÷ 44 = 7.14) which, to the nearest round number, is 7.

Answer B is incorrect: 12. This answer is incorrect as the number of employees working for organisations with a turnover in excess of £1M (535.5) has been divided by the number of other organisations (44), instead of dividing the remaining number of employees (314.5) by 44.

Answer C is incorrect: 15. This answer is incorrect as the number of remaining employees (314.5) has been divided by the number of organisations with a turnover in excess of £1M (21).

Answer D is incorrect: 19. This answer is incorrect as it has taken the total number of employees (850) and divided by the number of other organisations (44).

Answer E is incorrect: 26. This answer is incorrect as the number of employees working for organisations with a turnover in excess of £1M (535.5) has been divided by the number of those organisations (21).

Question 13

Less than, less than or equal to, greater than, greater than or equal to: rule
- Less than *n* does not include *n*.
- Less than or equal to *n* does include *n*.
- Greater than *n* does not include *n*.
- Greater than or equal to *n* does include *n*.

Answer E is correct: 21.

Rationale
Step 1: check what is being asked. Here we need to find all the shop buildings less than 5 m high.

Step 2: the third group includes the heights 4–4.9 m. The fourth group includes the heights 5–5.9 m. We are only concerned with the shop buildings less than 5 m high so we do not include heights equalling 5 m or more.

Step 3: remember to count all the shop buildings less than 5 m high – so that is all the shop buildings in the first three groups, which is 3 + 6 + 12 = 21.

Step 4: therefore there are 21 shop buildings less than 5 m high.

Answer A is incorrect: 6. This is the amount of shop buildings in the group of heights 3–3.9 m only. Therefore this answer is incorrect as we also need to include the shop buildings in the groups 2–2.9 m and 4–4.9 m.

Answer B is incorrect: 9. This is the amount of shop buildings in the groups of heights 2–2.9 m and 3–3.9 m only. Therefore the answer is incorrect as we also need to include the shop buildings in the group 4–4.9 m.

Answer C is incorrect: 12. This is the amount of shop buildings in the group of heights 4–4.9 m only. Therefore the answer is incorrect as we also need to include the heights of shop buildings in the groups 2–2.9 m and 3–3.9 m.

Answer D is incorrect: 15. This is the sum of shop buildings in the groups of heights 2–2.9 m and 4–4.9 m. Therefore the answer is incorrect as we also need to include the heights of shop buildings in the group 3–3.9 m.

Question 14

Percentages: rule
To express one number as a **percentage** of another, write the first number as a fraction of the second and convert the fraction to a percentage by multiplying it by 100.

Answer C is correct: Less than 4 metres high.

Rationale

This can be found by deducing that all the other options cannot be possible. To check the calculation:

Step 1: count the number of shop buildings in the first two groups that are less than 4 m, which is 9.

Step 2: there are 45 shop buildings in total, so $9 \div 45 \times 100 = 20\%$ ($9 \div 45 = \frac{1}{5}$, which is the same as 20%).

Step 3: therefore it can be said that 20% of the shop buildings are less than 4 m high.

Answer A is incorrect: At least 5 metres high. 24 shop buildings are at least 5 m high, which is not 20% as $24 \div 45$ is approximately 50%.

Answer B is incorrect: At least 3 metres and less than 6 metres high. 33 of the shop buildings are at least 3 m high and less than 6 m high, which is not 20% as $33 \div 45$ is approximately 75%.

Answer D is incorrect: Less than 5 metres high. 21 of the shop buildings are less than 5 m high, which is not 20% as $21 \div 45$ is approximately 46%.

Answer E is incorrect: At least 7 metres high. Two of the shop buildings are at least 7 m high, which is not 20% as $2 \div 45$ is approximately 5%.

Question 15

Fractions: rule

To find one number as a **fraction** of another, you write the numbers as a fraction, with the first number on the top and the second number on the bottom. The top line of a fraction is called the numerator and the bottom line of a fraction is called the denominator.

Answer A is correct: $\frac{1}{3}$.

Rationale

Step 1: there are a total of 45 buildings, so this number goes on the bottom as the denominator.

Step 2: there are 15 buildings in the group 5–5.9 m, so this number goes on the top as the numerator.

Step 3: the fraction is therefore $\frac{15}{45}$.

Step 4: this can be reduced down, as both the top and bottom can be divided by 15, so $15 \div 45 = \frac{1}{3}$.

Step 5: therefore $\frac{1}{3}$ of the shop buildings are between 5 and 5.9 m high.

Answer B is incorrect: $\frac{1}{2}$. Half of 45 is 22.5, so this can be immediately dismissed.

Answer C is incorrect: $\frac{1}{4}$. One quarter of 45 is approximately 11, so this option is too low.

Answer D is incorrect: $\frac{3}{8}$. We know the denominator is 45 and this cannot be divided exactly by 8, so this cannot be the correct option.

Answer E is incorrect: $\frac{3}{4}$. We know the denominator is 45 and this cannot be divided exactly by 4, so this cannot be the correct option.

Question 16

Ratio: rule
A **ratio** allows one quantity to be compared with another quantity. Any two numbers can be compared by writing them alongside each other with the numbers separated by a ratio sign (:).

Answer B is correct: 4:5.

Rationale
Step 1: the total number of shop buildings less than 5 m is the original number plus the number of new shop buildings: 3 + 6 + 12 + 4 + 7 = 32.

Step 2: the total number of shop buildings 5 m and above is the original number plus the number of new shop buildings: 15 + 7 + 2 + 5 + 7 + 4 = 40.

Step 3: write the figures separated by the ratio sign with the lower number being compared first, so here 32:40.

Step 4: reduce these figures down if possible. In this instance both can be divided by 8 to give 4:5.

Answer A is incorrect: 3:4. Multiplying both sides of this ratio by 8 gives 24:32 and so this option cannot be correct, as the ratio is 32:40.

Answer C is incorrect: 5:6. Multiplying both sides of this ratio by 8 gives 40:48 and so this option cannot be correct, as the ratio is 32:40.

Answer D is incorrect: 5:8. Multiplying both sides of this ratio by 8 gives 40:64 and so this option cannot be correct, as the ratio is 32:40.

Answer E is incorrect: 7:10. Multiplying both sides of this ratio by 8 gives 56:80 and so this option cannot be correct, as the ratio is 32:40.

Question 17

Interpreting data: rule

When **interpreting data**, this may involve identifying information presented in some form of pictorial or visual display.

Answer A is correct: One too few.

Rationale

Step 1: add the total amount of biscuit varieties in the first table, which is 19.

Step 2: add together the values in each group in the second table, which is 5 + 3 + 5 + 1 + 4 = 18.

Step 3: 19 − 18 = 1. Therefore there is one variety of biscuit omitted from the second table.

Answer B is incorrect: Two too few. There is only one variety of biscuit missing from the second table.

Answer C is incorrect: One too many. There is one variety of biscuit missing from the second table, not one too many.

Answer D is incorrect: Two too many. There is one variety of biscuit missing from the second table, not two too many.

Answer E is incorrect: Total number of brands correct. There is a variety of biscuit omitted from the second table – therefore this statement is incorrect.

Question 18

Interpreting data: rule

When **interpreting data**, this may involve identifying information presented in some form of pictorial or visual display.

Answer E is correct: 2.25 g.

Rationale

Step 1: for digestives, 5 packets weigh 150 × 5 = 750 g. Divide by 100 = 7.5. Therefore total fat is 7.5 × 4.2 = 31.50 g.

Step 2: for shortbreads, 5 packets weigh 130 × 5 = 650 g. Divide by 100 = 6.5. Therefore total fat is 6.5 × 4.5 = 29.25 g.

Step 3: therefore the difference in fat between the two types of biscuits is 31.50 − 29.25 = 2.25 g.

Answer A is incorrect: 0.3 g. This answer is the difference between the fat content of 100 g of digestives (4.2 g) and the fat content of 100 g of shortbreads (4.5 g), i.e. 4.5 − 4.2 = 0.3 g.

Answer B is incorrect: 1.5 g. In this answer the fat content for digestives has been multiplied by 5 instead of 7.5, as has the fat content for shortbreads (i.e. 4.5 × 5 = 22.5, 4.2 × 5 = 21 and 22.5 − 21 = 1.5 g). However, the fat content is given in amounts per 100 g and so the total weight of biscuits must be calculated first.

Answer C is incorrect: 1.75 g. This answer is simply a miscalculation of the figures.

Answer D is incorrect: 2.05 g. Again, this answer is simply a miscalculation of the figures.

Question 19

Median: rule
The **median** of a distribution is the middle value when the values are arranged in order. When there are two middle values (i.e. for an even number of values), you add the two middle numbers and divide by 2.

Answer D is correct: Rearrange the numbers into numerical order and then find the tenth number.

Rationale
The median of a distribution is the middle value when the values are arranged in order. In the table there are 19 separate values and therefore the tenth value is the median.

Answer A is incorrect: Find the tenth number and divide this by 2. Here there is an odd number of values, so there is no need to divide anything by 2, only find the middle value.

Answer B is incorrect: Add all the numbers together and divide by 19. This is the method for finding the mean, not the median.

Answer C is incorrect: Find the average and divide by 2. This is not a method for finding any type of average.

Answer E is incorrect: Find the fat content figure that occurs most frequently. This is the method for finding the mode, not the median.

Question 20

Substitution: rule
Substitution means that you replace the letters in a formula or expression by the given number.

Answer A is correct: $X = 25 \dfrac{G}{(28.3)}$

Rationale

Step 1: we are converting to ounces (X) – i.e. finding what the equivalent ounces are – therefore X is on the left of the equals sign.

Step 2: we are told that grams are divided by 28.3. Therefore the equation so far is $\dfrac{G}{28.3}$

Step 3: finally we are told that $\dfrac{G}{28.3}$ must be multiplied by 25, so the formula is now $X = 25 \dfrac{G}{(28.3)}$

Answer B is incorrect: $G = \dfrac{25X}{(28.3)}$. This is incorrect as it has the G on the left side but it is not grams that are being calculated. We do not need to check the remainder of the equation.

Answer C is incorrect: $G = \dfrac{25}{28.3X}$. Again this is not correct as it has the G on the left side so we do not have to check the remainder of the equation.

Answer D is incorrect: $X = 28.3 \dfrac{G}{(25)}$. Here the 28.3 and the 25 are the wrong way round as we must divide G by 28.3 and then multiply the whole thing by 25.

Answer E is incorrect: $X = \dfrac{28.3}{(25G)}$. This is incorrect as G must be divided by 28.3 and not the other way round, and 25 is a multiplication not division factor.

Question 21

Addition (decimals): rule
To **add** two or more numbers containing decimals the sum can be done as an ordinary addition or, as with 'multiplication of decimals', you can ignore the decimal point. However, for addition you only count the number of digits after the decimal point for one of the numbers.

Answer C is correct: £10.90.

Rationale
In using ordinary addition the numbers are summed, £3.20 (one sausage and mash) + £3.50 (one fish and chips) + £3.00 (one vegetarian pancake) + £1.20 (portion of chips), i.e. 3.20 + 3.50 + 3.00 + 1.20 = £10.90.

Alternatively, you can ignore the decimal point, i.e. 320 + 350 + 300 + 120 = 1090, then replace the decimal point to give £10.90.

Answer A is incorrect: £7.90. This answer has only summed 3.20 + 3.50 + 1.20 = 7.90 and has not included the £3.00 for a vegetarian pancake.

Answer B is incorrect: £9.70. This answer has only summed 3.20 + 3.50 + 3.00 = £9.70 and has not included the £1.20 for a portion of chips.

Answer D is incorrect: £12.10. This answer has summed 3.20 + 3.50 + 3.00 + 1.20 + 1.20 = £12.10, having included an extra £1.20 for an additional portion of chips.

Answer E is incorrect: £7.40. This answer has only summed 3.20 + 3.00 + 1.20 = 7.40 and has not included the £3.50 for one sausage and mash.

Question 22

Addition and subtraction: rule
To **add** two or more numbers containing decimals the sum can be done as an ordinary addition or, as with 'multiplication of decimals', you can ignore the decimal point. However, for addition you only count the number of digits after the decimal point for one of the numbers.

To **subtract** take away one value from another value.

Answer B is correct: £4.80.

Rationale
Step 1: In using ordinary addition the numbers are summed, £4.45 (All Day Breakfast) + £0.75 (coffee), i.e. 4.45 + 0.75 = £5.20.

Alternatively, if you ignore the decimal point, i.e. 445 + 75 = 520, then replace the decimal point to give £5.20.

Step 2: Then subtract £5.20 from £10.00, i.e. £10.00 − £5.20 = £4.80.

Answer A is incorrect: £4.50. This has assumed the addition to sum £5.50, i.e. £10 − £5.50 = £4.50.

Answer C is incorrect: £5.80. This has assumed the addition to sum £4.20, i.e. £10 − £4.20 = £5.80.

Answer D is incorrect: £6.20. This has assumed the addition to sum £3.80, i.e. £10 − £3.80 = £6.20.

Answer E is incorrect: £5.20. This is the value of the sum, not the change.

Question 23

Range: rule

The **range** of a distribution is found by working out the difference between the highest value and the lowest value. The range should always be given as a single value.

Answer C is correct: £1.45.

Rationale

Step 1: the highest value is £4.45.

Step 2: the lowest value is £3.00.

Step 3: the range = £4.45 – £3.00 = £1.45.

Step 4: the range of the prices of food is £1.45.

Answer A is incorrect: 95p. For this to be correct, if the highest value in the distribution was £4.45 then the lowest value would have to be £3.50, i.e. £4.45 – £3.50 = 95p. Alternatively, if the lowest value in the distribution was £3.00 then the highest value would have to be £3.95, i.e. £3.95 – £3.00 = 95p.

Answer B is incorrect: £1.00. For this to be correct, if the highest value in the distribution was £4.45 then the lowest value would have to be £3.45, i.e. £4.45 – £3.45 = £1.00. Alternatively, if the lowest value in the distribution was £3.00 then the highest value would have to be £4.00, i.e. £4.00 – £3.00 = £1.00.

Answer D is incorrect: £1.55. For this to be correct, if the highest value in the distribution was £4.45 then the lowest value would have to be £2.90, i.e. £4.45 – £2.90 = £1.55. Alternatively, if the lowest value in the distribution was £3.00 then the highest value would have to be £4.55, i.e. £4.55 – £3.00 = £1.55.

Answer E is incorrect: £3.00. For this to be correct, if the highest value in the distribution was £4.45 then the lowest value would have to be £1.45, i.e. £4.45 –£1.45 = £3.00. Alternatively, if the lowest value in the distribution was £3.00 then the highest value would have to be £6.00, i.e. £6.00 – £3.00 = £3.00.

Question 24

Percentages (fraction): rule

To change a **fraction** to a **percentage** you multiply by 100.

Answer E is correct: 20%.

Rationale

Step 1: find the number of fish that weigh 1.9 kg or less; this = 5.

Step 2: the fraction of fish that Bob threw back into the river is therefore $\frac{5}{25}$ that can be reduced to $\frac{1}{5}$ by dividing the numerator and denominator by 5.

Step 3: to change the fraction to a percentage, multiply it by 100, i.e. $\frac{1}{5} \times 100$ = 20%.

Step 4: Bob threw 20% of the fish back into the river.

Answer A is incorrect: 16%. For this to be correct Bob would have needed to throw 4 fish back into the river, i.e. $\frac{4}{25} \times 100 = 16\%$.

Answer B is incorrect: 32%. For this to be correct Bob would have needed to throw 8 fish back into the river, i.e. $\frac{8}{25} \times 100 = 32\%$.

Answer C is incorrect: 40%. For this to be correct Bob would have needed to throw 10 fish back into the river, i.e. $\frac{10}{25} \times 100 = 40\%$.

Answer D is incorrect: 60%. For this to be correct Bob would have needed to throw 15 fish back into the river, i.e. $\frac{15}{25} \times 100 = 60\%$.

Question 25

Fractions: rule

To find one number as a **fraction** of another, you write the numbers as a fraction, with the first number on the top and the second number on the bottom. The top line of a fraction is called a numerator and the bottom line of a fraction is called the denominator.

Answer D is correct: $\frac{4}{5}$.

Rationale

Step 1: the number of fish that weigh 2.9 kg or less = 20 (numerator).

Step 2: the total number of fish = 25 (denominator).

Step 3: write the number as a fraction, i.e. $\frac{20}{25}$. This fraction can be reduced by dividing the numerator and denominator by 5 to give $\frac{4}{5}$.

Step 4: Bob threw $\frac{4}{5}$ of the fish he caught back into the river.

Answer A is incorrect: $\frac{1}{2}$. This must be incorrect as the denominator, i.e. the total number of fish, is 25 and this is not divisible by 2 to provide this answer.

Answer B is incorrect: $\frac{2}{3}$. This must be incorrect as the denominator, i.e. the total number of fish, is 25 and this is not divisible by 3 to provide this answer.

Answer C is incorrect: $\frac{3}{4}$. This must be incorrect as the denominator, i.e. the total number of fish, is 25 and this is not divisible by 4 to provide this answer.

Answer E is incorrect: $\frac{1}{3}$. This must be incorrect as the denominator, i.e. the total number of fish, is 25 and this is not divisible by 3 to provide this answer.

Question 26

Ratios: rule
A **ratio** allows one quantity to be compared to another quantity. Any two numbers can be compared by writing them alongside each other with the numbers being separated by a ratio sign (:).

Answer A is correct: 1:4.

Rationale
Step 1: there is no need to approximate figures on this occasion as they are clearly provided, i.e. 5 (fish thrown back) and 25 (total number of fish caught).

Step 2: if there were 5 fish thrown back then 20 were not thrown back, i.e. 25 − 5 = 20.

Step 3: write these figures separated by the ratio sign with the number being compared first, so here 5:20.

Step 4: reduce these figures if possible. Both can be divided by 5 to give a ratio of 1:4.

Step 5: the ratio of the fish that Bob threw back into the river compared with those he did not is 1:4.

Answer B is incorrect: 1:3. We know the first number of the ratio is 5 (fish thrown back). Therefore the second number of the ratio for this answer would be 5 × 3 = 15 (fish not thrown back), to give 5:15 or 1:3.

Answer C is incorrect: 2:5. We know 5 fish were thrown back so the first number of the ratio is 5 × 2 = 10. The second number of the ratio for this answer would be 25 (5 × 5), to give 10:25 or 2:5.

Answer D is incorrect: 2:3. We know 5 fish were thrown back so the first number of the ratio is 5 × 2 = 10. The second number of the ratio for this answer would be 15 (5 × 3), to give 10:15 or 2:3.

Answer E is incorrect: 1:5. We know 5 fish were thrown back so the first number of the ratio is 5 x 1 = 5. The second number of the ratio for this answer would be 25 (5 × 5), to give 5:25 or 1:5.

Question 27

Percentages: rule
To express one number as a **percentage** of another, write the first number as a fraction of the second and convert the fraction to a percentage by multiplying it by 100.

Answer B is correct: 35%.

Rationale
Step 1: count the number of batteries lasting less than 4 hours (do not include ones lasting 4 hours or more), which = 7.

Step 2: 7 as a fraction of 20 (the total number of batteries) = $\frac{7}{20}$.

Step 3: convert to a percentage so $\frac{7}{20} \times 100 = 35\%$.

This can be calculated without a calculator. To get 20 (the denominator) to 100 it must be multiplied by 5 so the numerator, which is 7, must also be multiplied by 5, which gives $7 \times 5 = 35$ or 35%.

Step 4: therefore the percentage of batteries lasting less than 4 hours is 35 per cent.

Answer A is incorrect: 25%. 25% is the same as $\frac{1}{4}$, and $\frac{1}{4}$ of 20 is 5, so this cannot be correct, as it is too low.

Answer C is incorrect: 55%. 55% is approximately half, and one half of 20 is 10, so this cannot be correct; as it is too high.

Answer D is incorrect: 65%. 65% is greater than a half and half of 20 is 10, so this cannot be correct, as it is much too high.

Answer E is incorrect: 20%. 20% is the same as $\frac{1}{5}$, and $\frac{1}{5}$ of 20 is 4, so this cannot be correct, as it is too low.

Question 28

Mode: rule
The **mode** is the number in the distribution that has the highest frequency, that is, it appears the most times in a collection of values.

Answer A is correct: 3.

Rationale
Looking at the table which relates to this question, the number that appears the most times in the range is 3; it appears 4 times.

Answer B is incorrect: 4. The number 4 only appears 3 times.

Answer C is incorrect: 4.5. The number 4.5 does not appear at all.

Answer D is incorrect: 6. The number 6 only appears 3 times.

Answer E is incorrect: 5. The number 5 only appears 3 times.

Question 29

Range: rule
The **range** of a distribution is found by working out the difference between the highest value and the lowest value. The range should always be given as a single value.

Answer B is correct: 8.

Rationale
The highest value in a list of battery life spans is 9 and the lowest value is 1 so the range of the distribution is $9 - 1 = 8$.

Answer A is incorrect: 1. This is the lowest value of the distribution; it is not the range.

Answer C is incorrect: 9. This is the highest value of the distribution; it is not the range.

Answer D is incorrect: 20. The range is the difference between 9 and 1 so this option can be immediately disregarded.

Answer E is incorrect: 10. The range is the difference between the highest and lowest values and the highest value is 9 not 10.

Question 30

Mean: rule
The **mean** (or arithmetic mean) of a distribution is found by summing the values of the distribution and dividing by the number of values.

Answer E is correct: 4.65.

Rationale
Step 1: add together to numbers of the values; $9 + 8 + 7 + 7 + 6 + 6 + 6 + 5 + 5 + 5 + 4 + 4 + 4 + 3 + 3 + 3 + 3 + 2 + 2 + 1 = 93$.

Step 2: divide the total by the number of values, which in this case is 20; $93 \div 20 = 4.65$.

This can be quickly calculated by dividing 93 by 2 instead of 20, which = 46.5, then move the decimal place one place to the left to take you back to the value of 20, which = 4.65.

Step 3: the mean of the batteries' life span is 4.65.

Answer A is incorrect: 3. This is the mode of the distribution; it is not the mean.

Answer B is incorrect: 8. This is the range of the distribution; it is not the mean.

Answer C is incorrect: 4.5. This is the median of the distribution; it is not the mean.

Answer D is incorrect: 9. This is the highest value of the distribution; it is not the mean.

Chapter 10
The Abstract Reasoning subtest

This chapter will help you to:

- understand the purpose and format of abstract reasoning tests
- prepare for the Abstract Reasoning subtest using general abstract reasoning questions
- test your knowledge and understanding of abstract reasoning-type questions
- identify those abstract reasoning skills where development is required.

Introduction

Pearson VUE describes the purpose of this subtest as follows: 'The Abstract Reasoning subtest assesses candidates' ability to infer relationships from information by convergent and divergent thinking.'

First, we will clarify what is generally meant by convergent and divergent thinking. These styles of thinking, or cognitive styles, were first identified and named by J.P. Guilford in the 1950s and have been extensively researched since. The following is a brief description of the two styles.

Convergent thinking

The problem-solving skills associated with convergent thinking are characterised by the tendency to focus on the one correct, or single best, solution to a problem. Therefore problems that have unique solutions lend themselves well to convergent thinking.

Divergent thinking

The problem-solving skills associated with divergent thinking are characterised by the ability to produce a number of novel ideas that are relevant to a particular problem. Therefore open-ended problems that do not have unique solutions lend themselves well to divergent thinking.

How are convergent and divergent thinking usually measured?

Convergent thinking is usually measured by conventional multi-choice questions that have unique correct answers (as in the Abstract Reasoning subtest). The measurement of divergent thinking attempts to tap more creative approaches by asking for more solutions to the problem, of which more than one answer could be correct.

The UKCAT claims for the Abstract Reasoning subtest are as follows:

> The items include irrelevant and distracting material which can lead the individual to unsatisfactory solutions. The non-critical person may remain satisfied with such solutions. The test therefore measures both an ability to change track, critically evaluate and to generate hypotheses which can be relevant in the development of new ideas and systems.

However, the format of the subtest does appear to be based on convergent thinking as each question has a unique correct answer.

You may be interested to know that research has found that convergers usually specialise in physical sciences, mathematics or classics, hold conventional attitudes and opinions, pursue technical or mechanical interests, and tend to be emotionally inhibited. Divergers, on the other hand, usually specialise in the arts or biology, hold unconventional attitudes and opinions, pursue interests involving interaction with others, and tend to be emotionally uninhibited. It has been suggested that divergent thinking is an essential prerequisite of exceptional intellectual performance. However, candidates for higher education have usually been selected on the basis of exam results, which generally tap convergent thinking, and the UKCAT appears to be the same.

What are abstract reasoning tests?

Abstract reasoning tests purport to measure 'general intelligence' or 'general intellectual reasoning ability'. General intelligence is supposedly our innate capacity to reason as opposed to our socially and educationally developed verbal and numerical reasoning capacity. Some argue that verbal and numerical reasoning tests can probe innate skills (as does the UKCAT), but there is a strong correlation between the results from GCSEs and A-levels with tests of aptitude. The arguments about intelligence theories are vast and, to some extent, have never been resolved. However, increasingly employers and educational institutions are using reasoning tests as selection measures. Therefore we need to attempt to 'level the playing field'.

Abstract reasoning tests attempt to measure how well you can solve problems from basic principles. To answer these types of questions, you need to identify the underlying logic. Abstract reasoning questions are usually presented in sequences of symbols, patterns or shapes arranged in squares or rows. Examples of these types of questions are in the 'Example questions' section of this chapter.

Typically, to answer these types of questions, you have to work through three stages.

Stage one

The identification of the symbols or shapes used and what they have in common. For example, the things to look for will be as follows:

■ *Number*: the number of symbols or shapes.

■ *Size*: do the shapes or symbols vary in size – small to large?

■ *Shape*: various symbols, circles, squares, triangles or other multi-sided or faceted shapes.

■ *Characteristics*: curved lines, straight lines, dotted lines, number or type of angles or points, open sides to shapes, divided shapes, shapes that can be drawn with or without removing the pencil from the paper or back tracking (for example, an X or a square).

■ *Colour*: colour may be used, but not usually; could be negative to positive (e.g. black to white or vice versa).

Stage two

The identification of the pattern that the symbols or shapes form:

■ *Repeating patterns*: the symbols repeated in twos, threes, fours, etc.

■ *Rotation*: the symbol or shape rotated clockwise or anti-clockwise.

■ *Mirror images*: are the symbols or shapes mirror images (e.g. flipped left to right or top to bottom)?

■ *Direction*: do the symbols or shapes move from top left, to top right, to bottom right, to bottom left, or do they move diagonally?

Stage three

Generally, this would be the identification of which symbol(s), shape(s), etc., form the next part of the sequence. In the case of the UKCAT Abstract Reasoning subtest it is the identification of whether the 'Test Shape' belongs with 'Set A', 'Set B' or 'Neither Set'. Therefore, you will need to use the processes described in stage one and stage two above to determine whether the test shape has the same characteristics as Set A, Set B or Neither Set.

Abstract Reasoning subtest

The Abstract Reasoning subtest is an onscreen test that will consist of 65 items associated with 13 pairs of Set A and Set B shapes. Five test shapes will be presented with each pair of Set A and Set B shapes, and there are three answer options for each test shape: Set A, Set B or Neither Set. Each test shape is presented with the pair of Set A and Set B shapes on a separate screen with the three answer options below. A period of 16 minutes is allowed for the subtest, with one minute for administration time and the remaining 15 minutes to answer the questions.

Before attempting the practice questions based on the approach taken in the UKCAT, you should find it beneficial to work through the following questions. The first examples are based on classic abstract reasoning questions with response options of 1–6 and progress through to the format used in the UKCAT using the response options of Set A, Set B or Neither Set.

The first three examples based on classic abstract reasoning items have just one question. Examples 4 and 5 relate to two sets of shapes (four boxes in each set) but with the same response format of the UKCAT. The final examples (6 and 7) are based on the UKCAT format and will serve as a 'trial run' prior to attempting the abstract reasoning practice test. This staged approach should develop your understanding of how this type of reasoning test is structured and should also develop your confidence and ability when answering the questions.

Sets of shapes and response formats

The sets of shapes are normally regular or irregular shapes and symbols which are usually black and white, but colour may be used. For the purpose of the UKCAT, the two sets of shapes (Set A and Set B) each contain six boxes. Each pair of sets will be followed by five test shapes which have to be matched to the response format of Set A, Set B or Neither Set. The example questions will clarify this.

Example questions

The following three examples require you to select the correct answer from the six options provided.

Example 1

What comes next?

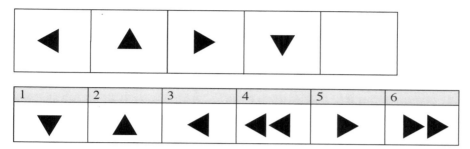

Rationale

Stage 1: the shapes in the question are all single, same-size, black triangles.

Stage 2: the triangles rotate clockwise by one turn.

Stage 3: the solution must be a single, black triangle; the triangle must rotate clockwise one more turn.

Distracters: options 1, 2 and 5 could be considered but can be eliminated, as there is not a logical pattern.

Irrelevant: options 4 and 6 can be eliminated immediately as logic points to a single black triangle.

The answer to Example 1 is 3. The triangle will be back in the original position.

Example 2

What comes next?

Rationale

Stage 1: the shapes in the question are all black, same-size clubs or diamonds; there are three groups of two shapes and one single shape.

Stage 2: the shapes are sequenced 2, 1, 2 and 2; the only repeat is the alternating two clubs in the same position.

Stage 3: the solution must be two clubs.

Distracters: options 1, 5 and 6 could be considered but can be eliminated, as there is no logical pattern.

Irrelevant: options 2 and 3 are diamonds and can be eliminated immediately as logic points to clubs.

The answer to Example 2 is 4. The two clubs are in the same position.

Example 3

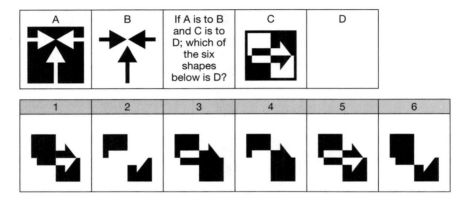

Rationale

Stage 1: the shapes in boxes A and B of the question are the same but B is the negative of A (e.g. white to black and black to white); the shape in box C is different from A and B.

Stage 2: the shape in box C must relate to box D using the same criteria as the relationship between A and B.

Stage 3: the solution must be a negative of C.

Distracters: all the other options are distracters but can be easily discounted when examined for change from black to white and vice versa.

Irrelevant: all options could have been relevant on the basis of shape.

The answer to Example 3 is 5. This is the negative of item C.

The following two examples use a format very similar to the UKCAT in that you have to match a test shape to Set A, Set B or Neither Set. However, in this staged approach we are using only four boxes in Set A and B as opposed to the six used in the UKCAT. The key point is, first, to determine what distinguishes each set to arrive at the rationale. Answering the associated questions should then be a relatively quick process as the test shapes will contain the key characteristics identified as belonging to Set A, Set B or Neither Set.

Examples 4 and 5

Set A

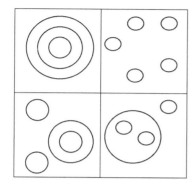

Set B

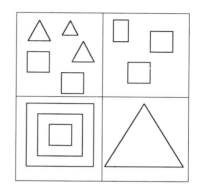

Example 4 Test Shape

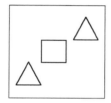

Example 5 Test Shape

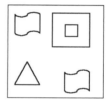

Rationale

Stage 1: the shapes in Set A are all circles, the shapes in Set B are triangles and/or squares; the size and number of the shapes vary in both sets; the shapes are all white in both sets; shapes can be within others in both sets; the shapes in Set A are all circular (curved lines), the shapes in Set B have straight lines only.

Stage 2: both sets contain no logical repeats, rotations, mirror images or direction changes.

Stage 3: therefore, the solution must be the Stage 1 characteristic of shapes with curved lines in Set A and shapes with straight lines in Set B. Any test shape containing both will belong with Neither Set.

Distracters: shapes, numbers of shapes and position of shapes (including shapes within others).

Irrelevant: two different shapes in Set B.

The answer to Example 4 is Set B. The test shape belongs to Set B as all the shapes have straight lines.

The answer to Example 5 is Neither Set. The test shape belongs to Neither Set as two of the shapes have both straight and curved lines.

The following examples are based on the UKCAT format.

Examples 6 and 7

Set A   Set B

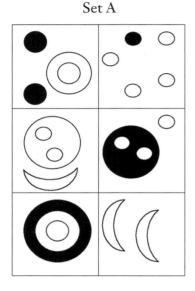   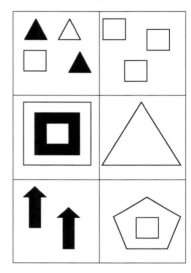

Example 6 Test Shape   Example 7 Test Shape

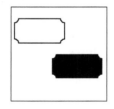   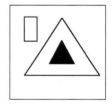

Rationale

Stage 1: the shapes in Set A include circles, ovals and ellipses; the shapes in Set B include diamonds, triangles, squares, rectangles and arrows; the size and number of the shapes vary in both sets; the shapes are white, black or black and white in both sets; shapes can be within others in Set A; the shapes in Set A all have curved lines, the shapes in Set B all have straight lines.

Stage 2: both sets contain no logical repeats, rotations, mirror images or direction changes.

Stage 3: therefore, the solution must be the Stage 1 characteristic of shapes with curved lines in Set A and shapes with straight lines in Set B. Any test shape containing both will belong with Neither Set.

Distracters: shapes, numbers of shapes, position of shapes and shapes within others.

Irrelevant: different shapes in both sets and use of black.

The answer to Example 6 is Neither Set. The test shape belongs to Neither Set as the shapes have both straight and curved lines.

The answer to Example 7 is Set B. The test shape belongs to Set B as the shapes all have straight lines.

Abstract Reasoning practice subtest

For the purpose of this book the practice subtest is just over three-quarters the length of the UKCAT subtest. Also, the five test shapes related to each of the seven 'Sets' will be displayed on the same page.

The Abstract Reasoning practice subtest provided below contains 50 items associated with ten pairs of shapes (Set A and Set B). The shapes in Set A are related in some way, as are the shapes in Set B, but the sets are not related to each other. Following each pair of sets there are five test shapes (questions). Examine Set A and Set B using the stages described in the introductory section, and decide whether each individual test shape belongs to Set A, Set B or Neither Set.

If you want to simulate 'test conditions', you are advised to use rough paper to mark down your choice for each of the questions (i.e. Set A, Set B or Neither Set). You should aim to complete the test within *13 minutes* (i.e. just over three-quarters the time allowed for the actual subtest).

The correct answer and rationale to each of the questions are produced in the section following the practice subtest.

Questions 1 to 5

Set A   Set B

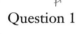

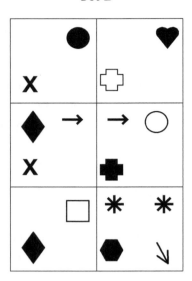

Question 1	Question 2	**Test Shapes**	Question 4	Question 5

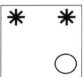 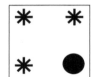 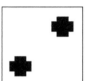 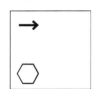

Questions 6 to 10

Set A   Set B

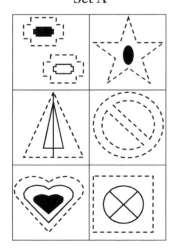   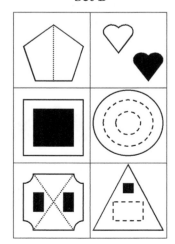

Test Shapes

Question 6 ᵇ   Question 7 ₐ   Question 8 ᵇ   Question 9 ᵇ   Question 10 ₙ

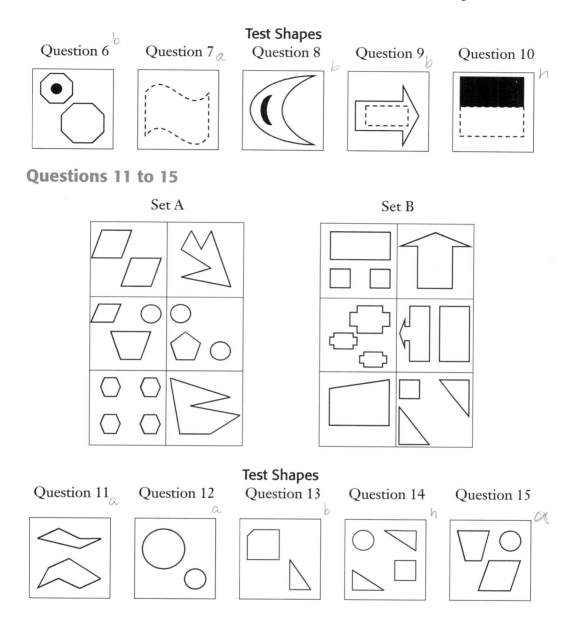

Questions 11 to 15

Set A   Set B

Test Shapes

Question 11 ₐ   Question 12 ₐ   Question 13 ᵇ   Question 14 ₙ   Question 15 ₐₑ

Questions 16 to 20

<table>
<tr><td align="center">Set A</td><td align="center">Set B</td></tr>
</table>

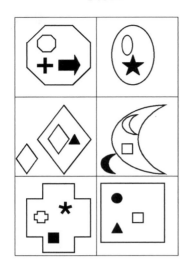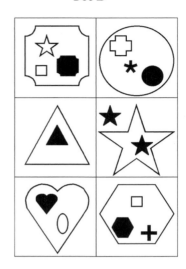

Test Shapes

Question 16	Question 17	Question 18	Question 19	Question 20

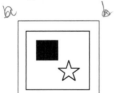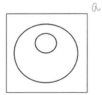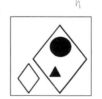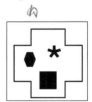

Questions 21 to 25

<table>
<tr><td align="center">Set A</td><td align="center">Set B</td></tr>
</table>

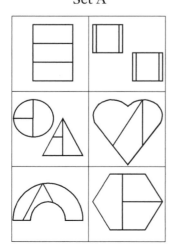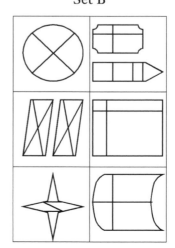

Test Shapes

Question 21	Question 22	Question 23	Question 24	Question 25
n	*a*	*b*	*n*	*a*

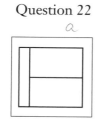 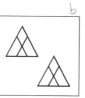 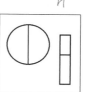 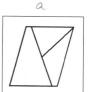

Questions 26 to 30

Set A

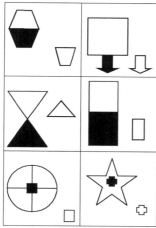

Set B

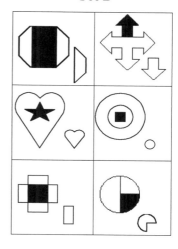

Test Shapes

Question 26	Question 27	Question 28	Question 29	Question 30
h	*b*	*a*	*n*	*a*

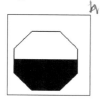 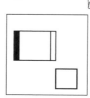 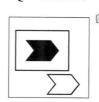 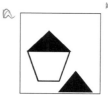 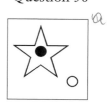

Questions 31 to 35

Set A

Set B

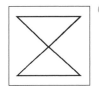   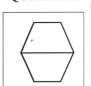

Test Shapes

Question 31   Question 32   Question 33   Question 34   Question 35

Questions 36 to 40

Set A

Set B

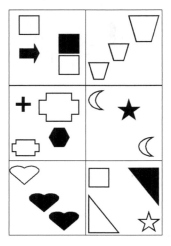

Test Shapes

Question 36   Question 37   Question 38   Question 39   Question 40

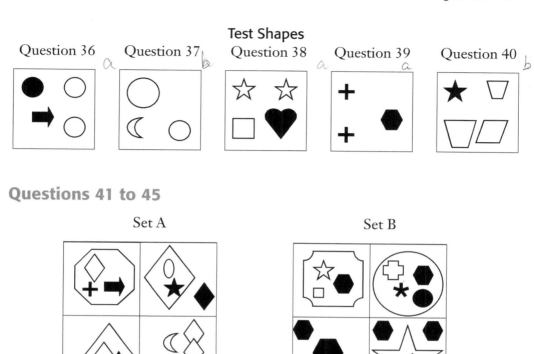

Questions 41 to 45

Set A   Set B

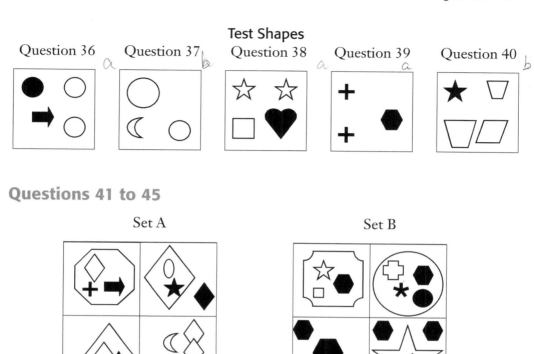

Test Shapes

Question 41   Question 42   Question 43   Question 44   Question 45

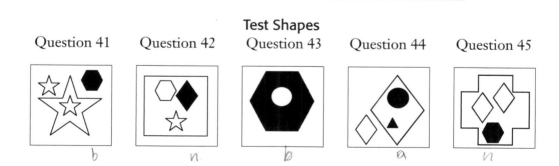

Questions 46 to 50

Set A   Set B

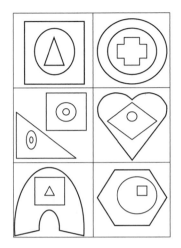 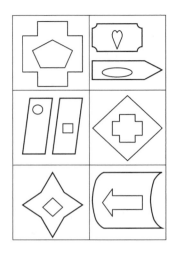

Test Shapes

| Question 46 | Question 47 | Question 48 | Question 49 | Question 50 |

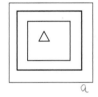 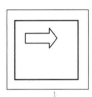 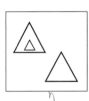 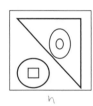 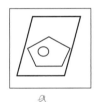

a   b   n   n   a

Abstract Reasoning practice subtest: answers

Question number	Correct response	Question number	Correct response
1	Set A	26	Neither Set
2	Set B	27	Set B
3	Neither Set	28	Set A
4	Neither Set	29	Neither Set
5	Set A	30	Set A
6	Set B	31	Set A
7	Set A	32	Set B
8	Set B	33	Set A
9	Set B	34	Set B
10	Neither Set	35	Set A
11	Set A	36	Neither Set
12	Set A	37	Set B
13	Set B	38	Set A
14	Neither Set	39	Set A
15	Set A	40	Set B
16	Set A	41	Set B
17	Set B	42	Neither Set
18	Set A	43	Set B
19	Neither Set	44	Set A
20	Neither Set	45	Neither Set
21	Neither Set	46	Set A
22	Set A	47	Set B
23	Set B	48	Neither Set
24	Neither Set	49	Neither Set
25	Set A	50	Set A

Abstract Reasoning practice subtest: explanation of answers

Questions 1 to 5

Rationale

Stage 1: the shapes and symbols in Set A include a cross, diamond, hexagon, 'X' and a heart, and arrows, squares, asterisks and circles; the shapes and symbols in Set B include a heart, square and a hexagon, and circles, 'X's', crosses, diamonds, arrows and asterisks; the size of the shapes is the same in both sets; the number of shapes varies in both sets; the shapes are white or black both sets, but there are more black shapes in Set B.

Stage 2: both sets contain no rotations, mirror images or direction changes; however, both sets contain a logical repeat: in Set A all the boxes contain at least one white shape and in Set B all the boxes contain one black shape; these shapes are not repeated in any box in either set; Set A has one box containing two shapes but these are different and, therefore, there is still a logical repeat of one white shape.

Stage 3: therefore, the solution must be the Stage 2 characteristic of an unrepeated white shape in each box in Set A and an unrepeated black shape in each box in Set B. Any test shape not meeting the criteria belongs to Neither Set.

Distracters: shapes, symbols, numbers of shapes and symbols, position of shapes and two white shapes in one of the boxes in Set A.

Irrelevant: different shapes and symbols in both sets.

Answer to question 1 is Set A: the test shape belongs to Set A as it contains a white shape.

Answer to question 2 is Set B: the test shape belongs to Set B as it contains a black shape.

Answer to question 3 is Neither Set: the test shape belongs to Neither Set as it does not contain any shapes, only symbols.

Answer to question 4 is Neither Set: the test shape belongs to Neither Set as the two black shapes are the same and this does not meet the Stage 2 requirement of a black shape that is not repeated in the box.

Answer to question 5 is Set A: the test shape belongs Set A as it contains a white shape.

Questions 6 to 10

Rationale

Stage 1: the shapes in Set A include a star, square and an oval, and crosses, triangles, circles, semi-circles and hearts; the shapes in Set B include a pentagon, plaque and a triangle, and hearts, squares, circles and rectangles; the size and number of the shapes vary in both sets; the shapes are white, black or black and white in both sets; shapes can be within others in both sets; the shapes have curved and straight lines in both sets; the outlines of all the shapes in Set A are broken and the outlines of all the shapes in Set B are solid.

Stage 2: both sets contain no logical repeats, rotations, mirror images or direction changes.

Stage 3: therefore, the solution must be the Stage 1 characteristic of shapes with external broken outlines in Set A and shapes with external solid outlines in Set B. Any test shape not meeting the criteria belongs to Neither Set.

Distracters: shapes, numbers of shapes, position of shapes; shapes within others.

Irrelevant: the use of dotted or solid lines within the shapes.

Answer to question 6 is Set B: the test shape belongs to Set B as the two shapes have solid outlines.

Answer to question 7 is Set A: the test shape belongs to Set A as the shape has a broken outline.

Answer to question 8 is Set B: the test shape belongs to Set B as the outer shape has a solid outline.

Answer to question 9 is Set B: the test shape belongs to Set B as the outer shape has a solid outline.

Answer to question 10 is Neither Set: the test shape belongs to Neither Set as it has both a broken and solid outline.

Questions 11 to 15

Rationale

Stage 1: the shapes in Set A include a trapezium and a pentagon, and rhombuses, irregular shapes, circles and hexagons; the shapes in Set B include a quadrilateral, and rectangles, squares, arrows, crosses and triangles; the size and number of the shapes vary in both sets; the shapes are all white in both sets; the shapes in Set A do no contain any right angles; the shapes in Set B all have some right angles.

Stage 2: both sets contain no logical repeats, rotations, mirror images or direction changes.

Stage 3: therefore, the solution must be the Stage 1 characteristic of shapes with no right angles in Set A and shapes with at least one right angle in Set B. Any test shape not meeting the criteria belongs to Neither Set.

Distracters: shapes, numbers of shapes and the position of shapes.

Irrelevant: the use of other angles in Set B.

Answer to question 11 is Set A: the test shape belongs to Set A as the two shapes do not contain any right angles.

Answer to question 12 is Set A: the test shape belongs to Set A as the two circles do not contain any right angles.

Answer to question 13 is Set B: the test shape belongs to Set B as the two shapes contain one or more right angles.

Answer to question 14 is Neither Set: the test shape belongs to Neither Set, even though three of the shapes contain right angles. The circle does not contain any right angles and, to meet the criteria, all the shapes must contain at least one right angle.

Answer to question 15 is Set A: the test shape belongs to Set A as the three shapes do not contain any right angles.

Questions 16 to 20

Rationale
Stage 1: the shapes and symbols in Set A include a plus sign, arrow, star, asterisk, triangle and a circle, and hexagons, ovals, diamonds, ellipses, crosses and squares; the shapes and symbols in Set B include a cross, asterisk, oval and a plus sign, and stars, plaques, squares, circles, triangles, hearts and hexagons; the size and number of the shapes vary in both sets; the shapes are white, black or black and white in both sets; shapes can be within others in both sets; the shapes have curved and straight lines in both sets.

Stage 2: both sets contain no rotations, mirror images or direction changes; there is a logical repeat in each set: the larger outline shapes in Set A are reflected as a smaller image within the shape in each box; the larger outline shapes in Set B are reflected as a smaller negative (black) image within the shape in each box.

Stage 3: therefore, the solution must be the Stage 2 characteristic of the large shape being reflected as a smaller image within the shape in Set A and the large shape being reflected as a smaller negative (black) image with the shape in Set B. Any test shape not meeting the criteria belongs to Neither Set.

Distracters: smaller shapes outside larger shapes and number of shapes.

Irrelevant: different shapes and symbols.

Answer to question 16 is Set A: the test shape belongs to Set A as the larger star has a smaller star within.

Answer to question 17 is Set B: the test shape belongs to Set B as the larger square has a smaller negative (black) square within.

Answer to question 18 is Set A: the test shape belongs to Set A as the larger circle has a smaller circle within.

Answer to question 19 is Neither Set: the test shape belongs to Neither Set as the larger diamond is not reflected within as either a smaller white or negative image.

Answer to question 20 is Neither Set: the test shape belongs to Neither Set as the larger cross is not reflected within as either a smaller white or negative image.

Questions 21 to 25

Rationale
Stage 1: the shapes in Set A include a rectangle, circle, triangle, heart, 'half donut' and a hexagon, and squares; the shapes in Set B include a circle, plaque, square and a star, and arrows and parallelograms; the size and number of the shapes vary in both sets; the shapes are all white in both sets; the individual shapes within the boxes are divided into three in Set A and the individual shapes within the boxes are divided into four in Set B.

Stage 2: both sets contain no logical repeats, rotations, mirror images or direction changes.

Stage 3: therefore, the solution must be the Stage 1 characteristic of individual shapes being divided into three and four in Set A and Set B, respectively. Any test shape not meeting the criteria belongs to Neither Set.

Distracters: shapes, numbers of shapes and position of shapes.

Irrelevant: differing shapes within each set.

Answer to question 21 is Neither Set: the test shape belongs to Neither Set as the circle has been divided into six.

Answer to question 22 is Set A: the test shape belongs to Set A as the square has been divided into three.

Answer to question 23 is Set B: the test shape belongs to Set B as the two individual triangles have been divided into four.

Answer to question 24 is Neither Set: the test shape belongs to Neither Set as the circle and the rectangle have been divided into two.

Answer to question 25 is Set A: the test shape belongs to Set A as the parallelogram has been divided into three.

Questions 26 to 30

Rationale

Stage 1: the shapes in Set A include a hexagon, trapezium, circle and a star, and squares, arrows, triangles, rectangles and crosses; the shapes in Set B include an octagon, trapezium, star and three quarters of a circle, and rectangles, arrows, hearts, circles and squares; the size and number of the shapes vary in both sets; the shapes are white, black or black and white in both sets; shapes can be within others in both sets.

Stage 2: both sets contain no rotations, mirror images or direction changes; both sets contain logical repeats: in Set A the black part of the large shape is reflected separately as a white shape which may differ in size; in Set B the separate shape does not reflect the black part of the large shape but it is still white.

Stage 3: therefore, the solution must be the Stage 2 characteristic of the black part of the larger shape being reflected as a separate white shape in Set A and the black part of the larger shape not being reflected in the smaller white shape in Set B. Any test shape not meeting the criteria belongs to Neither Set.

Distracters: shapes, numbers of shapes, position of shapes, shapes within others and the repeat of part of the shapes in Set B.

Irrelevant: differing shapes in both sets.

Answer to question 26 is Neither Set: the test shape belongs to Neither Set as there is not a smaller white shape.

Answer to question 27 is Set B: the test shape belongs to Set B as the black rectangular part of the large shape is not reflected in the smaller white shape.

Answer to question 28 is Set A: the test shape belongs to Set A as the black arrow within the larger shape is reflected in the smaller white shape.

Answer to question 29 is Neither Set: the test shape belongs to Neither Set as the black triangle from the larger shape is reflected as a smaller black image, not white.

Answer to question 30 is Set A: the test shape belongs to Set A as the black circle within the star is reflected in the smaller white shape.

Questions 31 to 35

Rationale

Stage 1: the shapes and symbols in Set A include a lightning flash, heart, hexagon, triangle, cross and a bracket; the shapes and symbols in Set B include a circle, diamond, square, plaque, 'X' and a 'no' symbol; the size and number of the shapes are equal in both sets; the shapes are white or lines only in both sets; the shapes in Set A can all be drawn without lifting the pen or pencil off the paper; the shapes in Set B have intersecting lines or lines within which means they cannot be drawn without back tracking or lifting the pen or pencil off the paper.

Stage 2: both sets contain no logical repeats, rotations, mirror images or direction changes.

Stage 3: therefore, the solution must be the Stage 1 characteristic shapes that can be drawn without lifting the pen or pencil off the paper, as in Set A; or shapes that cannot be drawn without back tracking or lifting the pen or pencil off the paper, as in Set B. Therefore, by definition, all test shapes will meet the criteria for either Set A or Set B.

Distracters: shapes, and single intersecting lines when within shapes as in question 35.

Irrelevant: differing shapes in both sets.

Answer to question 31 is Set A: the test shape belongs to Set A as it can be drawn from any point without lifting the pen or pencil off the paper.

Answer to question 32 is Set B: the test shape belongs to Set B as the two adjoining brackets cannot be drawn from any point without lifting the pen or pencil off the paper.

Answer to question 33 is Set A: the test shape belongs to Set A as it can be drawn from any point without lifting the pen or pencil off the paper.

Answer to question 34 is Set B: the test shape belongs to Set B as the addition of two lines (or legs) to the trapezium means it cannot be drawn from any point without lifting the pen or pencil off the paper.

Answer to question 35 is Set A: the test shape belongs to Set A as it can be drawn without lifting the pen or pencil off the paper, providing you start from either end of the middle or intersecting line.

Questions 36 to 40

Rationale

Stage 1: the shapes in Set A include a heart, triangle and a crescent, and cylinders, circles, squares, stars and hexagons; the shapes in Set B include an arrow, a cross, and squares, trapeziums, plaques, crescents, stars, hearts and triangles; the size of the shapes vary a little in both sets; the number of shapes varies in both sets; the shapes are white or black in both sets, but there are more black shapes in Set A.

Stage 2: the arrow in Set A rotates to the right and changes to black and the black triangle in Set B rotates twice to the right and changes to white, but this does not constitute a logical pattern in either set; however, there is a logical repeat in each set: in Set A all the boxes contain at least two shapes the same irrespective of size or colour; in addition, the two shapes are either positioned vertically or horizontally to each other and can be left, middle or right, or top middle or bottom, respectively; in Set B the minimum matching two shapes are diagonally opposite on either diagonal; these features are unique to each set and a test shape cannot contain both; in addition the two shapes have to be on the outer edges or corners of the boxes.

Stage 3: therefore, the solution must be, in part, a Stage 1 characteristic, in that the shapes can vary in size and can be black or white; and, in part, the Stage 2 characteristic of vertical or horizontal positioning of two shapes in each box in Set A and diagonal positioning of two shapes in each box in Set B. Any test shape not meeting the criteria belongs to Neither Set.

Distracters: numbers of shapes, colours of shapes, rotations and sizes of shapes.

Irrelevant: different shapes in both sets.

Answer to question 36 is Neither Set: the test shape belongs to Neither Set as it has both horizontal and diagonal lines of at least two circles therefore it contains characteristics of both sets.

Answer to question 37 is Set B: the test shape belongs to Set B as it contains a diagonal line of circles.

Answer to question 38 is Set A: the test shape belongs to Set A as it contains a horizontal line of stars.

Answer to question 39 is Set A: the test shape belongs to Set A as it contains a vertical line of crosses.

Answer to question 40 is Set B: the test shape belongs Set B as it contains a diagonal line of trapeziums.

Questions 41 to 45

Rationale

Stage 1: the shapes and symbols in Set A include an oval, arrow and a star, hexagon and a circle, and diamonds, crosses, triangles, crescents and squares; the shapes and symbols in Set B include a plaque, heart and an asterisk and an oval, and stars, squares, hexagons and circles; the size of the shapes varies in both sets; the number of shapes varies in both sets; the shapes are white or black in both sets, but there are more black shapes in Set B.

Stage 2: both sets contain no rotations, mirror images or direction changes; however, both sets contain a logical repeat: in Set A all the boxes contain at least one white diamond and in Set B all the boxes contain at least one black hexagon; the shapes can overlap or touch in either set; Set A has one box containing overlapping shapes and Set B has one box containing touching shapes; Set B has one box which only contains hexagons but this is irrelevant.

Stage 3: therefore, the solution must be the Stage 2 characteristic of at least one white diamond in each box in Set A and at least one black hexagon in each box in Set B. Any test shape not meeting the criteria belongs to Neither Set.

Distracters: symbols, numbers of shapes and symbols, position of shapes and size of shapes.

Irrelevant: overlapping or touching shapes and the same shape in one box in Set B.

Answer to question 41 is Set B: the test shape belongs to Set B as it contains at least one black hexagon.

Answer to question 42 is Neither Set: the test shape belongs to Neither Set as it contains a white hexagon and a black diamond which are both the wrong colour shapes for either set.

Answer to question 43 is Set B: the test shape belongs to Set B as it contains at least one black hexagon.

Answer to question 44 is Set A: the test shape belongs to Set A as it contains at least one white diamond.

Answer to question 45 is Neither Set: the test shape belongs to Neither Set as it contains at least one white diamond and one black hexagon, therefore it has the characteristics of both sets.

Questions 46 to 50

Rationale

Stage 1: the shapes and symbols in Set A include a cross, heart, diamond, horseshoe and a hexagon, and squares, circles, triangles and ovals; the shapes and symbols in Set B include a pentagon, heart, circle, square, star and an oval, and plaques, arrows, parallelograms, crosses, and diamonds; the size of the shapes varies in both sets; the number of shapes varies in both sets; the shapes are white in both sets, but there are more shapes in Set A.

Stage 2: both sets contain no rotations, mirror images or direction changes; however, both sets contain a logical repeat: in Set A all the boxes contain at least one white shape which contains two more white shapes within each other and in Set B all the boxes contain at least one white shape which has one more white shape within it; this is still a logical repeat even when the boxes contain more than one cluster of shapes.

Stage 3: therefore, the solution must be the Stage 2 characteristic of one white shape which contains two more white shapes within each other in Set A and one white shape which has one more white shape within it in Set B. Any test shape not meeting the criteria belongs to Neither Set.

Distracters: shapes and the number of groupings of shapes.

Irrelevant: different shapes in both sets.

Answer to question 46 is Set A: the test shape belongs to Set A as it contains a white shape which contains two more white shapes within each other.

Answer to question 47 is Set B: the test shape belongs to Set B as it contains a white shape which has one more white shape within it.

Answer to question 48 is Neither Set: the test shape belongs to Neither Set as one of the white shapes does not contain another shape.

Answer to question 49 is Neither Set: the test shape belongs to Neither Set as one white shape contains one other shape and the second white shape contains two more white shapes, therefore this test shape has the characteristics of both sets.

Answer to question 50 is Set A: the test shape belongs to Set A as it contains a white shape which contains two more white shapes within each other.

Chapter 11
The Decision Analysis subtest

This chapter will help you to:

- understand the purpose and the format of the Decision Analysis subtest
- prepare for the Decision Analysis subtest using general decision analysis questions
- test your knowledge and understanding of decision analysis-type questions
- identify those decision analysis skills where development is required.

Introduction

Pearson VUE describes the purpose of this subtest as follows:

> The Decision Analysis subtest assesses candidates' ability to decipher and make sense of coded information. You will be presented with a scenario and a significant amount of information together with items that become progressively more complex and ambiguous. The judgements that are required cannot be based on logical deduction alone and this simulates the realities of real-world decision-making where decisions cannot always be made with all the information neatly accessible in one place.

What are decision analysis tests?

Decision analysis tests are, as their name suggests, a measure of an individual's quality of decision-making, both in respect of the adequacy of the decision and the promptness with which the decision has been taken. The behavioural indicators implicit within decision analysis include the ability to identify the relevant information, analyse the facts and consider all the issues, promptness in making the decisions and basing decisions on a reasoned consideration of the evidence.

Decision analysis often forms part of a number of dimensions being assessed in the recruitment process and in other types of selection and, in particular, for situations requiring managerial skills. The dimensions can be assessed either through a series of exercises and scenarios or by the use of psychometric tests. However, the use of such tests specifically to determine an individual's ability to make decisions is unusual.

Decision Analysis subtest

The Decision Analysis subtest is an onscreen test that will consist of one scenario and 26 items associated with that scenario. The scenario may contain text, tables and other types of information. This subtest differs from the other UKCAT subtests in that the 26 items will have four or five response options and, for some items, more than one of the options may be correct. Where more than one of the response options is required, this should be clearly identified within the item. A period of 30 minutes is allowed for the subtest, with one minute for administration time and the remaining 29 minutes to answer the questions.

Before attempting the practice questions based on the approach taken in the UKCAT, you should find it beneficial to work through the following questions. The scenario and items have been formatted along the lines to be used in the UKCAT, and the answers and the rationales for the correct answers follow each question.

Scenario, response formats and example questions

The scenario for a decision analysis test can contain information in a variety of formats. However, in view of the time constraints imposed for this subtest, it is probable that the information contained in the scenario will be reasonably short and specific, and is likely to include an initial paragraph of explanatory text, a list of codes in tabular or similar format and a couple of worked examples. New information will added at some stage during the test to add to the complexity of the items. This will be in the form of additional codes with a brief explanation. The information and examples will be accessible throughout the test.

The scenario provided by the Pearson VUE website, in their practice test, has an explanatory paragraph followed by information in a tabular format to which new information is added for the final example. The practice test information consists of a series of codes from which the items have been taken. Essentially, this requires the respondent to identify the words contained within part of the code and to see which answer options best fits those particular words.

The explanatory paragraph directs the respondent to make 'your best judgement' in selecting the correct option or options. 'Best judgement' means your judgement based solely on the codes themselves and not on what you might consider to be reasonable. This is not dissimilar to the Verbal Reasoning subtest in that you need to focus on the information provided and not use your knowledge or experience in answering any of the items.

Codes may be combined to produce a new but related concept (for example, the codes of 'air' and 'ice' could combine to become 'snow'). In addition, you will be asked to make more subtle judgements, particularly when the ordering of the codes is not obvious or when some codes appear to be missing.

In line with the Pearson VUE format for the Decision Analysis subtest, the scenarios used both in the example below and in the following practice test are in the style of coded information. Where appropriate, the requirement of selecting more than one option is clearly identified.

Example questions

The following examples are intended to go from the simple to the complex, commencing with a simple code and building into codes with both specific and additional information, increasing the level of complexity.

Example scenario 1

A group of explorers in the Amazon rain forest stumble upon what appears to be the ruined site of an ancient civilisation. In exploring one of the ruined buildings, they find a tablet of stone with what appears to be a coded message. What does it mean?

100504E   50O5ES   65050A

This coded message can be answered by changing the numbers to roman numerals to reveal the meaning:

CLIVE LOVES VILLA

This example is used to introduce you to the world of cryptography (codes and ciphers) where use is often made of cryptograms (i.e. coded messages). However, you will be pleased to hear that the UKCAT does not require you to break a code or cipher. The scenario will provide you with both the code and its meaning. Although this sounds simple, it is not quite so – particularly when you are under time pressure to make prompt decisions. We'll therefore look at a scenario and items similar to those used in the UKCAT.

Example scenario 2

Counter-intelligence codes

In the secret world of counter-intelligence it is not unusual for messages between agencies and agents to be encrypted. In the modern era this encryption can be extremely sophisticated but, for the purposes of this scenario, a method of letter, number and symbol substitution is used. The codes used by one counter-intelligence agency within Europe are presented in the table below. The information from the codes may not always be complete, but you are asked to make your best judgement based on this information and not on what you might consider to be reasonable.

Table: counter-intelligence codes

Operating codes	Routine codes
α = delay	01 = explosive
β = previous	02 = today
γ = cancel	03 = sun
δ = negative	04 = rain
ε = increase	05 = agent
ζ = hot	06 = public
η = opposite	07 = smoke
θ = include	08 = safe
	09 = building
	10 = drop
	11 = tonight
	12 = dark
	13 = weapon
	14 = abort
	15 = secret
	16 = operation

Below are two examples of how the codes work.

Example item 1

Examine the following coded message:

α, 16, 03, 04

The code combines the words 'delay', 'operation', 'sun', 'rain'.

Now examine the following sentences and try to determine which is the most likely interpretation of the code:

A. The operation is delayed due to sun and rain.
B. The operation is delayed due to sun.
C. The operation is delayed due to rain.
D. Delay the operation until it is dry.
E. Delay operation rainbow.

All the options contain elements of the codes. However, a decision has to be made as to which of the options provides the most likely interpretation.

Answer and rationale

Option E 'Delay operation rainbow' is the correct answer as it uses all the codes. Note 'sun' and 'rain' combine to make 'rainbow'.

Option A uses all the codes but it is not likely that the operation would be delayed for 'sun' and 'rain'. Look for a better option.

Option B does not use the code 'rain'.

Option C does not use the code 'sun'.

Option D introduces the word 'dry', which could relate to 'sun', but it does not use the code 'rain'.

Example item 2

Examine the following coded message:

06, 09, $\epsilon(08\eta)$, 11

The code combines the words 'public', 'building', 'increase (safe opposite)', 'tonight'.

Now examine the following sentences and try to determine which is the most likely interpretation of the code:

A. The public building is safe tonight.
B. The public building is dangerous.
C. People in the cinema are very safe tonight.
D. People in the building are in extreme danger today.
E. People in the cinema are in extreme danger tonight.

All the options contain elements of the codes. However, a decision has to be made as to which of the options provides the most likely interpretation.

Answer and rationale

Option E 'People in the cinema are in extreme danger tonight' is the correct answer as it uses all the codes. 'Public' can be 'people', a 'cinema' is a 'building', 'extreme danger' is an 'increase of the opposite of safe'.

Option A does not 'increase the opposite of safe'.

Option B does not use the word 'tonight' and it does not increase 'danger'.

Option C increases 'safe' rather than the 'opposite of safe'.

Option D introduces the code 'today', which is not used.

The following two examples will include new information, as detailed below:

NEW INFORMATION ADDED

Codes for specialisms and personality traits.

The Head of Counter-intelligence has appointed new agents and they use a more sophisticated coding system that will impact on the previous codes.

Specialist codes	Personality codes
A = full B = wound C = mortal D = fast E = enjoyable	101 = emotional 102 = assertive 103 = trusting 104 = confident 105 = practical 106 = volatile

---

Counter-intelligence codes

In the secret world of counter-intelligence it is not unusual for messages between agencies and agents to be encrypted. In the modern era this encryption can be extremely sophisticated but, for the purposes of this scenario, a method of letter, number and symbol substitution is used. The codes used by one counter-intelligence agency within Europe are presented in the table below. The information from the codes may not always be complete, but you are asked to make your best judgement based on this information and not on what you might consider to be reasonable.

Table: counter-intelligence codes

Operating codes	Routine codes	Specialist codes	Personality codes
α = delay β = previous γ = cancel δ = negative ε = increase ζ = hot η = opposite θ = include	01 = explosive 02 = today 03 = sun 04 = rain 05 = agent 06 = public 07 = smoke 08 = safe 09 = building 10 = drop	A = full B = wound C = mortal D = fast E = enjoyable	101 = emotional 102 = assertive 103 = trusting 104 = confident 105 = practical 106 = volatile

	11 = tonight 12 = dark 13 = weapon 14 = abort 15 = secret 16 = operation		

The following example has the codes in a different order from the solution.

Example item 3

Examine the following coded message:

101η, 101, 05, 102, 06, 106

The code combines the words 'emotional opposite', 'emotional', 'agent', 'assertive', 'public', 'volatile'.

Now examine the following sentences and try to determine which is the most likely interpretation of the code:

A. Agents are assertive and volatile with the public.
B. The public are calm in volatile situations.
C. People react in an emotionally volatile way with assertive agents.
D. Agents need to be assertive and emotional when dealing with calm people.
E. Agents need to be assertive and calm when dealing with emotionally volatile people.

All the options contain elements of the codes. However, a decision has to be made as to which of the options provides the most likely interpretation.

Answer and rationale
Option E 'Agents need to be assertive and calm when dealing with emotionally volatile people' is the correct answer as it uses all the codes. 'Public' can be 'people', 'calm' is the 'opposite of emotional'.

Option A does not use 'emotional opposite' (calm) or 'emotional'.

Option B does not use the words 'agent' and 'assertive'.

Option C does not use 'emotional opposite' (calm).

Option D is possible as it uses all the codes, but it is not the most likely solution. Look for a better option.

The following example has two options that could be correct and also has some information missing. When you sit the UKCAT you may not be aware that information is missing, but an analysis of the options should make this obvious. You are required to make a logical decision as to what the missing information is.

Example item 4

Examine the following coded message:

Dε, 16, 15, 05, 08, 11

The code combines the words 'fast increase', 'operation', 'secret', 'agent', 'safe', 'tonight'.

Now examine the following sentences and try to determine which is the most likely interpretation of the code:

A. A fast operation will ensure the safety of the public.
B. The secret agent will operate faster.
C. The secret agent is safe tonight following the operation.
D. The agent will have to carry out tonight's secret mission very quickly to ensure the safety of the public.
E. The agent will have to carry out tonight's secret operation very fast to ensure the building is safe.

All the options contain elements of the codes. However, a decision has to be made as to which of the options provides the most likely interpretation.

Answer and rationale

Options D and E could both be correct. Option D 'The agent will have to carry out tonight's secret mission very quickly to ensure the safety of the public' uses all the codes with the addition of the missing information 'public'. The word 'operation' can be 'mission' and 'very fast' can be 'very quickly'. Option E 'The agent will have to carry out tonight's secret operation very fast to ensure the building is safe' uses all the codes with the addition of the missing information 'building'.

Option A includes the addition of the missing information 'public' but it does not increase 'fast' and it does not use the words 'agent' and 'tonight'.

Option B cannot be discounted because it does not add in any missing information, but it can be discounted because it does not use the words 'safe' and 'tonight'.

Option C cannot be discounted because it does not add in any missing information, but it can be discounted because it does not use the word 'fast' increase.

Decision Analysis practice subtest

For the purpose of this book the practice subtest is just over half the length of the UKCAT subtest.

The Decision Analysis practice subtest provided below contains 21 items associated with one scenario that includes an introductory paragraph with coded information in a tabular format. The coded information is increased after question 8, and the items become more complex, as per the items in the example section above.

If you want to simulate 'test conditions', you are advised to use rough paper to mark down your choice for each of the questions (i.e. A, B, C, D or E). For questions with more than one answer option you will need to note all the appropriate options. You should aim to complete the test within 24 minutes (i.e. 6 minutes less than the time allowed for the actual subtest).

The correct answer and rationale to each of the questions are produced in the section following the practice subtest.

Decision Analysis practice subtest: questions

Intergalatic Space Agency codes

The Intergalatic Space Agency (ISA) is a highly expert team of code breakers. Their main remit is the interception of alien communications in the interests of universal security within the known solar system. In order to meet their undertakings, they are required to identify and decipher all intergalactic communications. The ISA are recruiting new agents and have set the following codes as their application test. To pass this test you will be required to interpret the coded questions and select the best option or options from those listed. The information from the codes may not always be complete, but you are asked to make your 'best judgement' based on this information and not on what you might consider to be reasonable.

Table: Intergalatic Space Agency codes

Operating codes	Basic codes
T = opposite U = negative V = unite W = hot X = enlarge Y = slow Z = similar	⚲ = me ☆ = others ◆ = oxygen ♣ = hydrogen ❤ = fire ▲ = Mars ◖ = Moon ✷ = Sun ✚ = tonight □ = home ◉ = see → = ship ■ = heavy ? = hard ✔ = prefer

Below are two examples of how the codes work.

Example item 1

Examine the following coded message:

✳, XW, ↟, ?, 👁

The code combines the words 'sun', 'enlarge hot', 'me', 'hard', 'see'.

Now examine the following sentences and try to determine which is the most likely interpretation of the code:

A. The sun is very large and is blinding me.
B. The very hot sun is burning me.
C. I like to see hot sunny weather.
D. The hot sun makes me squint.
E. The sun is very hot and I find it hard to see.

All the options contain elements of the codes. However, a decision has to be made as to which of the options provides the most likely interpretation.

Answer and rationale

Option E 'The sun is very hot and I find it hard to see' is the correct answer as it uses all the codes. Note 'me' can be 'I' and 'enlarge hot' is 'very hot'.

Option A uses 'hard' and 'see', which could combine to make 'blinding', but this option enlarges 'sun' and does not use the word 'hot'.

Option B introduces the word 'burning' and, although there is a code for 'fire', this is not included. In addition the code 'see' is missing.

Option C uses 'like' and 'weather', which are not code words. 'Sun' could become 'weather' but the code is not used twice.

Option D is almost possible, but 'hot' is not enlarged.

Example item 2

Examine the following coded message:

↟, X(U✔), ❤

The code combines the words 'me', 'enlarge (negative prefer)', 'fire'.

Now examine the following sentences and try to determine which is the most likely interpretation of the code:

A. I really like a fire.
B. I dislike sitting by the fire at home.

C. I am really fiery.
D. A big fire suits me.
E. I really dislike fire.

All the options contain elements of the codes. However, a decision has to be made as to which of the options provides the most likely interpretation.

Answer and rationale

Option E 'I really dislike fire' is the correct answer as it uses all the codes. 'Me' becomes 'I' and 'enlarge (negative prefer)' becomes 'really dislike'.

Option A uses 'enlarge prefer' instead of 'enlarge (negative prefer)' (dislike).

Option B introduces 'sitting', which is not a code, and 'home', which is not included.

Option C increases 'fire' and does not use 'negative prefer' (dislike).

Option D introduces the word 'big', which could be 'enlarge', but 'suits' is not the opposite of 'prefer'.

NEW INFORMATION ADDED	
Codes for technical aspects and personality traits.	
The ISA team has identified new codes that will impact on the previous codes.	
Technical codes	**Characteristic codes**
501 = warp	901 = warm
502 = damage	902 = sociable
503 = capacity	903 = aggression
504 = vacuum	904 = tense
505 = boost	905 = cynical
506 = aliens	

Intergalatic Space Agency codes

The Intergalatic Space Agency (ISA) is a highly expert team of code breakers. Their main remit is the interception of alien communications in the interests of universal security within the known solar system. In order to meet their undertakings, they are required to identify and decipher all intergalactic communications. The ISA are recruiting new agents and have set the following codes as their application test. To pass this test you will be required to interpret the coded questions and select the best option or options from those listed. The information from the codes may not always be complete, but you are asked to make your 'best judgement' based on this information and not on what you might consider to be reasonable.

Table: Intergalatic Space Agency codes

Operating codes	Basic codes	Technical codes	Characteristic codes
T = opposite U = negative V = unite W = hot X = enlarge Y = slow Z = similar	🏃 = me ☆ = others ◆ = oxygen ♣ = hydrogen ❤ = fire ▲ = Mars ◖ = Moon ☀ = Sun ✚ = tonight □ = home 👁 = see → = ship ■ = heavy ? = hard ✔ = prefer	501 = warp 502 = damage 503 = capacity 504 = vacuum 505 = boost 506 = aliens	901 = warm 902 = sociable 903 = aggression 904 = tense 905 = cynical

Question 1

What is the best interpretation of the following coded message: 🏃, ■T, Y, ◖

A.   Moon light shines on me.
B.   I am heavy and slow on the Moon.
C.   I am light and slow on the Moon.
D.   I am heavy and fast on the Moon.
E.   I am lighter than the Moon.

Question 2

What is the best interpretation of the following coded message: ♣X, V, ◆, ■X, ◆

A. Hydrogen combined with oxygen is heavier.
B. Hydrogen mixed with oxygen is heavy.
C. Water is largely oxygen.
D. Water is heavier than oxygen.
E. Hydrogen is a heavier gas than oxygen.

Question 3

What is the best interpretation of the following coded message: →, TY, □, ▲, ✚

A. The craft is fast and will get home from Mars tonight.
B. A fast ship will get me home from Mars.
C. A fast ship from Mars tonight.
D. A slow boat from Mars.
E. A fast ship will get to Mars tonight.

Question 4

What is the best interpretation of the following coded message: ⋏, ✔, ▲, U✔, ◖

A. I prefer the Moon to Mars.
B. I like Mars and the Moon.
C. The Moon and Mars have a negative effect on me.
D. I prefer Mars to the Moon.
E. Mars has no moons.

Question 5

What is the best interpretation of the following coded message: ?, ⋏, □, U□, ⋏

A. I find it hard being away from home.
B. I do not have a home.
C. It's hard for me to find a home.
D. Good homes are hard to locate.
E. I dislike my home.

Question 6

What is the best interpretation of the following coded message: ◖, V, X(U☐), ➔, ✚

A. The ship from the Moon will not reach home tonight.
B. The Moon craft is away from home tonight.
C. The craft is too far away from the Moon to reach tonight.
D. It is hard to reunite the ship with the Moon.
E. The ship is too far away to reach the Moon today.

Question 7

What is the best interpretation of the following coded message: U, T◆, ?, ☆, ✔, ◆, ▲

A. It is hard for the rest on Mars as there is no oxygen.
B. It is hard for us on Mars as we like air not carbon dioxide.
C. Carbon dioxide is preferred by people on Mars.
D. Martians prefer no oxygen.
E. No oxygen on Mars makes it hard for other people.

Question 8

What is the best interpretation of the following coded message: ➔, ❤, 502, W, ✳

A. Fires on the Sun damage ships.
B. Hot fires damage ships from the Sun.
C. Ships are built to resist damage from fire.
D. Craft suffer fire damage from the heat of the Sun.
E. Craft flying too close to the Sun get damaged.

Question 9

What is the best interpretation of the following coded message: 503, ➔, ☆, UY

A. Craft built to carry passengers go slower.
B. Passenger ships go fast.
C. Slow ships do not hold many people.
D. The ship is full of slow people.
E. An empty ship travels faster.

Question 10

What is the best interpretation of the following coded message: ♠, **?**, 902, 905, ☆

A. Cynical people find it hard to be sociable with me.
B. I am cynical of hard people.
C. I find it hard to be sociable with people who are cynical.
D. Other people are hard and cynical, not sociable like me.
E. I socialise with hard cynical friends.

Question 11

What is the best interpretation of the following coded message:
905, ♠, 901, ☆, 902, 506, 903, 904

A. Aliens are warm and sociable, while you and I are aggressive, tense and cynical.
B. We are aggressive and cynical when socialising with aliens.
C. Aliens have the same characteristics as you and I.
D. Aliens have the opposite characteristics to you and I.
E. We all have negative and positive characteristics.

Question 12

What is the best interpretation of the following coded message: ☆, 903, T✔, U, V☆
(NB: **Two** options are correct.)

A. Aggressive people are not liked in teams.
B. Teams like the opposition from aggressive people.
C. Teams do not like aggressive people.
D. No one likes aggressive teams.
E. People unite when faced with aggressive people.

Question 13

What is the best interpretation of the following coded message: 504, 501, X(TY)

A. A fast warp drive creates a vacuum.
B. The vacuum created by warp drive slows speed.
C. Speed in a vacuum will cause a twist.
D. A bigger warp creates a vacuum.
E. Warp drive creates a vacuum allowing increased speed.

Question 14

What is the best interpretation of the following coded message: 506, 902, 503, ⚹

A. I am sociable with aliens.
B. I have the capacity to be aggressive in dealing with aliens.
C. I need the ability to be sociable and aggressive in dealing with aliens.
D. Aliens do not have the capacity to be sociable and aggressive with me.
E. I have the same capacity of character as aliens.

Question 15

What is the best interpretation of the following coded message: ☆, 506, T903
(NB: **Two** options are correct.)

A. Other people make aliens aggressive.
B. Aliens are peace-loving people.
C. Aliens are gentle unlike other people.
D. Aliens are a non-aggressive race.
E. Others are aggressive to aliens.

Question 16

What is the best interpretation of the following coded message: ?TU, VT, 506, 506U
(NB: **Two** options are correct.)

A. It's not easy to separate aliens from non-aliens.
B. Aliens are hard and should be kept separate.
C. It's hard to separate aliens from non-aliens.
D. It's easy to unite aliens and non-aliens.
E. Aliens and non-aliens cannot be separated.

Question 17

What is the best interpretation of the following coded message: V, 905T, ➔, ☆U

A. Trust the others with the ship.
B. The others are cynical about uniting with the ship.
C. The others on the ship cannot be trusted.
D. Trust nobody with the ship.
E. The others will not be joining the ship.

Question 18

What is the best interpretation of the following coded message: ◆U, ▲, ◗, ✳, Z, XZU, WTW
(NB: **Two** options are correct.)

A. Oxygen levels and temperatures on Mars, the Sun and the Moon are similar.
B. Oxygen levels are similarly low on Mars, the Sun and the Moon but the temperatures vary greatly.
C. The lack of oxygen on Mars, the Sun and the Moon makes the temperatures vary.
D. Mars, the Sun and the Moon are very hot and devoid of oxygen.
E. The lack of oxygen on Mars, the Sun and the Moon is similar but the temperatures are very different.

Question 19

What is the best interpretation of the following coded message:
506U, 901, 902, 903, 904, 905, U, UT, YTY, ▲X

A. The moods of humans are influenced by Mars.
B. Negative and positive characteristics can be found in humans and aliens alike.
C. The movement of the planets has a positive or negative impact on human characteristics.
D. Human characteristics are opposite to aliens from Mars.
E. Fast moving planets influence human personality traits.

Question 20

What is the best interpretation of the following coded message: ⚲, 505, ◉, ◗■T, →, ⚲V☆, □
(NB: **Two** options are correct.)

A. It gives me a boost to see moonlight as the ship nears home.
B. We have to boost the ship to get from home to the Moon.
C. We can see moonlight at home from the ship.
D. I can see the moonlight as we boost the ship towards home.
E. The moonlight is visible to me as we boost the ship homewards.

Question 21

What is the best interpretation of the following coded message: ⚲V☆, ❤, 502, 904X, 501

A. The fire damage to the warp drive is a very tense situation for us.
B. We are very tense when we fire the warp drive.
C. Due to damage we cannot fire the warp drive.
D. We are very tense about the fire damage.
E. I am anxious about the damage to the warp drive.

Decision Analysis practice subtest: answers

Question number	Correct response
1	Option C
2	Option D
3	Option A
4	Option D
5	Option A
6	Option C
7	Option B
8	Option D
9	Option A
10	Option C
11	Option C
12	Options A & C
13	Option E
14	Option C
15	Options B & D
16	Options A & C
17	Option D
18	Options B & E
19	Option C
20	Options D & E
21	Option A

Decision Analysis practice subtest: explanation of answers

Question 1
Answer and rationale
🚶, ■T, Y, ◖

The code combines the words 'me', 'heavy opposite', 'slow', 'Moon'.

Option C 'I am light and slow on the Moon' is the correct answer as it uses all the codes. 'Me' becomes 'I' and 'opposite heavy' becomes 'light'.

Option A introduces the words 'light' and 'shines' and the code 'slow' is missing.
Option B has not used the 'opposite heavy' code to become 'light'.
Option D has not used the 'opposite heavy' code to become 'light'. Instead it has used the opposite of 'slow' to become 'fast'.
Option E has shown the 'opposite heavy' as 'lighter' and in addition has not used the code 'slow'.

Question 2
Answer and rationale
♣X, V, ◆, ■X, ◆

The code combines the words 'hydrogen enlarge', 'unite', 'oxygen', 'heavy enlarge', 'oxygen'.

Option D 'Water is heavier than oxygen' is the correct answer as it uses all the codes. 'Hydrogen enlarge' becomes 'H_2' and then 'unite' this with 'oxygen' becomes 'H_2O' – the chemical symbol for 'water'. The code 'heavy enlarge' becomes 'heavier' (than 'oxygen').

Option A has not 'enlarge(d) hydrogen' to 'H_2' and the final code 'oxygen' has not been included.
Option B has again not enlarged hydrogen to 'H_2'. In addition, 'heavy' has not been 'enlarge(d)' to 'heavier' nor is the final code 'oxygen' included.
Option C has identified 'H_2O' as water but has not included the code 'heavy enlarge'.
Option E has not 'enlarge(d) hydrogen' nor combined it with 'oxygen' to introduce the word 'water'.

Question 3
Answer and rationale
→, TY, □, ▲, ✚

The code combines the words 'ship', 'opposite slow', 'home', 'Mars', 'tonight'.

Option A 'The craft is fast and will get home from Mars tonight' is the correct answer as it uses all the codes, with 'opposite slow' becoming 'fast'.

Option B has used all the codes except for 'tonight'.
Option C has used all the codes except for 'home'.
Option D has not used 'opposite slow' to become 'fast'. It has used the word 'boat' where logically the word 'ship' would relate to 'spaceship' or possibly 'craft', and the code 'tonight' has not been included.
Option E has used all the codes except for 'home'.

Question 4
Answer and rationale
⋏, ✔, ▲, U✔, ◖

The code combines the words 'me', 'prefer', 'Mars', 'negative prefer', 'Moon'.

Option D 'I prefer Mars to the Moon' is the correct answer as it uses all the codes where the 'negative prefer' provides a negative preference to the Moon.

Option A has used all the codes but assigned the 'negative prefer' code to Mars and not the Moon.
Option B has used the word 'like' to 'prefer', which is acceptable, but ignored the 'negative prefer' to the Moon.
Option C has not used the code 'prefer' and has taken the code 'negative' out of context in relation to the assigned code 'prefer'.
Option E does not use the codes 'me', 'prefer' and 'Moon', although this is used in a different way by relating to 'moons'.

Question 5
Answer and rationale
?, ⚸, □, U□, ⚸

The code combines the words 'hard', 'me', 'home', 'negative home', 'me'.

Option A 'I find it hard being away from home' is the correct answer as it uses all the codes, with the first 'me' presented as 'I' and the second 'me' presented as 'being'. The 'negative home' is utilised by the word 'away'.

Option B does not use the code 'hard' and the second code of 'me'. The 'negative home' has been translated as 'do not have a home', which would require the code 'opposite' as opposed to 'negative'.

Option C does not use the second code of 'me' and has not used the code 'negative' in its association with 'home'. It has also introduced the word 'find'.

Option D does not use either of the codes 'me' and has not used the code 'negative' in association with 'home'. It has also introduced two words 'good' and 'locate'.

Option E does not use the code 'hard'. It has interpreted 'negative home' as 'dislike my home', which is a poor interpretation.

Question 6
Answer and rationale
◖, V, X(U□), →, ✚

The code combines the words 'Moon', 'unite', 'enlarge (negative home)', 'ship', 'tonight'.

Option C 'The craft is too far away from the Moon to reach tonight' is the correct answer as it uses all the codes. The words 'too far away' have been obtained from the code 'enlarge (negative home)', and 'reach' from code 'unite' (i.e. to reach the Moon tonight).

Option A uses all the codes but does not represent the logic of the codes, with the code 'home' being used in its context as opposed to its negative of 'away'.

Option B does not use the code 'unite' and again uses 'home' out of context of the codes.

Option D introduces a new code of 'hard' and does not use the code 'enlarge (negative home)'.

Option E does not use the code 'tonight' but introduces an unused code 'today'.

Question 7
Answer and rationale
U, T◆, ?, ☆, ✔, ◆, ▲

The code combines the words 'negative', 'opposite oxygen', 'hard', 'others', 'prefer', 'oxygen', 'Mars'.

Option B 'It is hard for us on Mars as we like air not carbon dioxide' is the correct answer as it uses all the codes. '…air not carbon dioxide' is found from the codes 'negative', 'opposite oxygen' and 'oxygen'. The code 'we' provides 'us' and the code 'prefer' provides 'like'.

Option A does not take into account the codes 'negative' and 'opposite oxygen'. It also ignores the code 'prefer'.
Option C does not use the code 'hard' and the repeated code 'oxygen'.
Option D does not use the codes 'hard' or 'others' and has interpreted 'negative', 'opposite oxygen' as 'no oxygen', which is incorrect. This answer also ignores the repeated 'oxygen' code and assumes the existence of 'Martians'.
Option E does not use the code 'prefer' or the second occurrence of 'oxygen'. It has assumed that the code 'negative' and 'opposite oxygen' is 'no oxygen' as opposed to carbon dioxide.

Question 8
Answer and rationale
→, ❤, 502, W, ✳

The code combines the words 'ship', 'fire', 'damage', 'hot', 'Sun'.

Option D 'Craft suffer fire damage from the heat of the Sun' is the correct answer as it uses all the codes. The word 'craft' has been correctly used in place of 'ship'.

Option A does not use the code 'hot'.
Option B does make use of all the codes but is not logical in its ordering. It would be difficult to justify an answer of ships coming from the Sun.
Option C does not use the codes 'hot' and 'Sun'.
Option E does not use the codes 'fire' and 'hot'.

Question 9
Answer and rationale
503, →, ☆, UY

The code combines the words 'capacity', 'ship', 'others', 'negative slow'.

Option A 'Craft built to carry passengers go slower' is the correct answer as it uses all the codes. The code 'capacity' is provided by 'carry' and 'others' by the word 'passengers'. 'Negative' in association with 'slow' means 'minus slow' in other words slower.

Option B does not use the code 'capacity', and 'fast' is the opposite of 'slow' and not the 'negative'.
Option C does contain all the codes but has not used the code 'negative slow' correctly and has also introduced the word 'many'.
Option D contains all the codes except the interpretation of the code 'negative slow'. In addition, this statement could not be seen as being logical as it is the ship and not the people who are slow.
Option E does not contain the code 'others', and the word 'empty' does not really fall within the definition of 'capacity'. In addition, 'faster' is the 'increased opposite' and not the negative of 'slow'.

Question 10
Answer and rationale
↑, ?, 902, 905, ☆

The code combines the words 'me', 'hard', 'sociable', 'cynical', 'others'.

Option C 'I find it hard to be sociable with people who are cynical' is the correct answer as it uses all the codes, with 'I' being used for the code 'me'.

Option A does use all the codes but, logically, Option C would be the preferred answer.
Option B does not include the code 'sociable'.
Option D does use all the codes but, logically, Option C would be the preferred answer.
Option E does use all the codes but, logically, Option C would be the preferred answer.

Question 11
Answer and rationale
905, ♠, 901, ☆, 902, 506, 903, 904

The code combines the words 'cynical', 'me', 'warm', 'others', 'sociable', 'aliens', 'aggression', 'tense'.

Option C 'Aliens have the same characteristics as you and I' is the correct answer as it uses all the codes. By using the word 'characteristics', the answer has combined the codes 'cynical', 'warm', 'sociable', 'aggression' and 'tense'.

Option A contains all the codes but has made decisions about assigning characteristic between 'aliens' and 'you and I' which is a subjective judgement.
Option B does not use the codes 'warm' and 'tense' or any collective term for their inclusion.
Option D does use all the codes but introduces the term 'opposite' which is not included.
Option E does not have the codes 'me' and 'aliens'. Even though 'me' might be construed as being part of 'we', the statement is general and may or may not include 'aliens'.

Question 12
Answer and rationale
☆, 903, T✔, U, V☆
(NB: **Two** options are correct.)

The code combines the words 'others', 'aggression', 'opposite prefer', 'negative', 'unite others'.

Option A 'Aggressive people are not liked in teams' and Option C 'Teams do not like aggressive people' are the correct answers as both contain all the codes. Options A and C have included 'not liked' and 'do not like', respectively, as part of the codes 'opposite prefer' and 'negative', and both have used 'teams' for the code 'unite others'.

Option B has not used the codes 'opposite prefer' and 'negative' in its use of the word 'like' and has misused the word 'opposition' from the code 'opposite'.
Option D has used the codes but the tenet of the statement does not reflect the way in which the codes are structured.
Option E does not use the codes 'opposite prefer' and 'negative'.

Question 13
Answer and rationale
504, 501, X(TY)

The code combines the words 'vacuum', 'warp', 'enlarge (opposite slow)'.

Option E 'Warp drive creates a vacuum allowing increased speed' is the correct answer as it contains all the codes. The words 'increased speed' reflect the code 'enlarge (opposite slow)'.

Option A includes all the codes but, in the way the codes are presented, Option E is judged to be a better answer.
Option B has not accounted for the code 'enlarge (opposite slow)' by using 'slows speed' instead of the opposite.
Option C has not used the code 'warp'.
Option D has not used the code 'enlarge (opposite slow)' correctly. It has interpreted this code as meaning 'bigger', which is not the opposite of 'slow'.

Question 14
Answer and rationale
506, 902, 503, ⚡

The code combines the words 'aliens', 'sociable', 'capacity', 'me'.

Option C 'I need the ability to be sociable and aggressive in dealing with aliens' is the correct answer even though it contains the word ' aggressive', which is not shown in the codes. This is an instance where you are being asked to make a more subtle judgement when some code(s) appear to be missing. In this instance it is necessary to consider carefully all the options before determining that this is the correct one.

Option A does not contain the code 'capacity' and can therefore be eliminated.
Option B does not contain the code 'sociable' though it has introduced another code 'aggression'. On the basis of it not containing one of the codes, it can be eliminated.
Option D contains all the codes but again has included another code 'aggression'. In addition, the option states 'do not have' and for this there would need to be some other 'negative' code. Because two new codes would be required as opposed to the one in Option C, this answer can be eliminated.
Option E is incorrect as it mentions 'character', which would include all the 'characteristics', and not just 'sociable' or even 'aggression'.

Question 15
Answer and rationale
✩, 506, T903
(NB: **Two** options are correct.)

The code combines the words 'others', 'aliens', 'opposite aggression'.

Option B 'Aliens are peace-loving people' and Option D 'Aliens are a non-aggressive race' are the correct answers. Both options contain all the codes and use appropriate terms for the codes 'opposite aggression' and 'others' – namely, 'peace-loving people' and 'non-aggressive race', respectively.

Option A does not take into account the code 'opposite aggression'.
Option C uses all the codes but adds further information that is not contained in the combinations (i.e. 'unlike other people').
Option E does not take into account the code 'opposite aggression'.

Question 16
Answer and rationale
?TU, VT, 506, 506U
(NB: **Two** options are correct.)

The code combines the words 'hard opposite (negative)', 'unite opposite', 'aliens', 'aliens negative'.

Option A 'It's not easy to separate aliens from non-aliens' and Option C 'It's hard to separate aliens from non-aliens' are the correct answers as both contain all the codes. Option A and Option C have interpreted 'hard opposite (negative)' as 'not easy' and 'hard' respectively, both of which could be correct.

Option B has not used the 'aliens negative' code to become 'non-aliens'.
Option D has not used the 'hard opposite (negative)' code to become 'not easy' or 'hard'. Instead it has used this code as 'easy'.
Option E has not used the code 'hard opposite (negative)' code to become 'not easy' or 'hard'. Instead it has introduced the word 'cannot'.

Question 17
Answer and rationale
V, 905T, →, ☆U

The code combines the words 'unite', 'cynical opposite', 'ship', 'others negative'.

Option D 'Trust nobody with the ship' is the correct answer as it uses all the codes. 'Unite' becomes 'with', 'cynical opposite' becomes 'trust' and 'others negative' becomes 'nobody'. Note, the codes do not have to be in the same order as the most logical interpretation.

Option A has not used the 'others negative' code to become 'nobody'. Instead it has used the 'others' code.
Option B has not used the 'others negative' code to become 'nobody'. Instead it has used the 'others' code. In addition, it has not used the 'cynical opposite' to become 'trust'. Instead it has used the 'cynical' code.
Option C has not used the 'others negative' code to become 'nobody'. Instead it has used the 'others' code.
Option E has not used the 'others negative' code to become 'nobody'. Instead it has used the 'others' code. In addition, it has used the 'unite' code as 'joining' instead of 'with'.

Question 18
Answer and rationale
◆U, ▲, ◗, ✳, Z, XZU, WTW
(NB: **Two** options are correct.)

The code combines the words 'oxygen negative', 'Mars', 'Moon', 'Sun', 'similar', '(enlarge) similar negative', 'hot opposite hot '.

Option B 'Oxygen levels are similarly low on Mars, the Sun and the Moon but the temperatures vary greatly' and Option E 'The lack of oxygen on Mars, the Sun and the Moon is similar but the temperatures are very different' are the correct answers as both contain all the codes. Options B and E have interpreted the 'oxygen negative' code as low levels of oxygen or a lack of oxygen, respectively, both of which could be correct. The code '(enlarge) similar negative' has been interpreted as 'vary greatly' or 'very different', again both of which could be correct. Both options have used the code 'hot opposite hot' as 'hot and cold' which in turn is interpreted as temperatures.

Option A has not used the code '(enlarge) similar negative' as 'vary greatly' or 'very different'. Instead it has used the code 'similar'.
Option C has associated the 'oxygen negative' code with the '(enlarge) similar negative' and the 'hot opposite hot' codes, which is a poor interpretation on the codes alone.
Option D has interpreted 'oxygen negative' as 'devoid of oxygen', which could be correct but it has not used the code 'hot opposite hot' as 'hot and cold' and in turn 'temperatures'. Instead it has used the code 'hot'.

Question 19

Answer and rationale

506U, 901, 902, 903, 904, 905, U, UT, YTY, ▲X

The code combines the words 'aliens negative', 'warm', 'sociable', 'aggression', 'tense', 'cynical', 'negative', 'negative opposite', 'slow opposite slow', 'Mars enlarge'.

Option C 'The movement of the planets has a positive or negative impact on human characteristics' is the correct answer as it uses all the codes. 'Slow opposite' becomes 'fast' and when combined with 'slow' this becomes movement. 'Mars enlarge' becomes 'planets', 'negative opposite' becomes 'positive' and the codes 'warm', 'sociable', 'aggression', 'tense' and 'cynical' are combined to become 'characteristics'. The word 'impact' is added and this is an instance where you are being asked to make a more subtle judgement when a code appears to be missing. It is necessary to consider carefully all the options before determining that this is the correct one.

Option A has not used the combined codes of 'slow opposite' (fast) and 'slow' to become movement. In addition the code 'enlarge Mars' has not been applied, neither have the codes 'negative' and 'negative opposite'. The word 'influenced' has been introduced which cannot be correct due to the other missing codes.
Option B has not used the combined codes of 'slow opposite' (fast) and 'slow' to become movement. In addition the code 'enlarge Mars' has not been applied. The code 'aliens' has been introduced along with other words, which cannot be correct due to the other missing codes.
Option D has applied 'opposite' to characteristics and has also omitted the codes of 'movement', negative and positive. In addition the code 'enlarge Mars' has not been applied.
Option E has not used the code 'slow' but would need to be considered carefully as, otherwise, it could be a plausible interpretation.

Question 20
Answer and rationale
⚤, 505, ☻, ▶■T, →, ⚤V☆, □
(NB: **Two** options are correct.)

The code combines the words 'me', 'boost', 'see', 'Moon heavy opposite', 'ship, 'me unite others', 'home'.

Option D 'I can see the moonlight as we boost the ship towards home' and Option E 'The moonlight is visible to me as we boost the ship homewards' are the correct answers as both contain all the codes. Option D has used the code 'me' as 'I' and has combined the codes 'Moon' and 'heavy opposite' (light) to become 'moonlight'. In addition it has used the codes 'me' 'unite' 'others' to become 'we'. Option E has just a couple of subtle differences in that it has used the code 'see' as 'visible' and has interpreted 'home' as 'homewards'.

Option A has not used the codes 'me', 'unite', others' to become 'we'.
Option B has not used the code 'me' and has not combined the code 'heavy opposite' (light) with Moon to become 'moonlight'.
Option C has not used the code 'me'.

Question 21
Answer and rationale
⚤V☆, ♥, 502, 904X, 501
The code combines the words 'me unite others', 'fire', 'damage', 'tense enlarge', 'warp'.

Option A 'The fire damage to the warp drive is a very tense situation for us' is the correct answer as it uses all the codes. The code 'warp' is interpreted as 'warp drive' and 'tense enlarge' becomes 'very tense'. In addition the codes 'me', 'unite', 'others' has become 'us'.

Option B has not used the code 'damage'.
Option C has not used the code 'tense enlarge' to become very tense.
Option D has not used the 'warp' as 'warp drive'.
Option E has used the code 'me' as 'I' and has not combined this with 'unite' 'others'. In addition it has used the word 'anxious', instead of 'tense', which could be correct but it has not been enlarged to 'very anxious'. The code 'fire' has also been omitted.

Chapter 12
The Non-Cognitive Analysis subtest

This chapter will help you to:

- understand the purpose and the format of the Non-Cognitive Analysis subtest
- prepare for the Non-Cognitive Analysis subtest using examples of non-cognitive analysis questions
- encourage the best approach when answering non-cognitive analysis questions.

Introduction

Pearson VUE describes the purpose of this subtest as follows:

The Non-Cognitive Analysis subtest assesses aspects of a candidate's empathy, integrity, honesty or robustness. Some questions will describe situations where candidates have to decide what to do according to their opinions or values. There are no right or wrong answers. Rather, candidates are asked to choose an answer from a series of options that most closely reflects their value system and what they believe is appropriate in each situation. Other questions cover a range of behaviours, attitudes, experiences, reactions to stress and feelings of well-being. Some of the questions are specifically designed to measure the degree of honesty with which the questionnaire has been approached.

What are Non-Cognitive Analysis tests?

The UKCAT Non-Cognitive Analysis subtest is basically a measure of an individual's personality in terms of their most likely traits (characteristics). Personality tests are generally formatted along similar lines in that they contain a range of statements that are rated according to one's own preferences, values and beliefs. They usually contain randomly mixed statements which load on to particular scales of personality, for example, 10 statements that would all load onto your level of 'anxiety', or 10 statements that would all load onto your level of 'empathy'. The robustness of these types of questionnaires is often dependent on having sufficient items for each scale; this will be discussed later in terms of the reliability and validity of these measures. It is not clear how many items and scales are actually contained in the UKCAT Non-Cognitive Analysis subtest. There are a large number of personality questionnaires available on the market, however, the majority are restricted to those who have been trained to use them.

The use of personality questionnaires in the commercial world as an aid to the recruitment, selection and development of staff has grown phenomenally over the last 20 years. Increasingly, organisations have realised that the levels of performance of staff with identical qualifications and skills differ greatly according to their 'personalities'. The consortium of universities using the UKCAT have introduced this type of assessment as an attempt to identify additional attributes and characteristics that it is believed do contribute to success in either medicine or dentistry careers; robustness, empathy and integrity.

The reliability and validity of personality questionnaires is limited. Test publishers should rigorously assess their questionnaires in order to arrive at a set of questions that best measure the intended scales (reliability) and these should then be validated against other measures of the same scales and more importantly external measures, for example, does your scale of integrity really relate to the level of integrity a person demonstrates in reality. In practice, the most rigorous measures available are not that great at actually predicting performance. For example, the very best measures of the scale of 'anxiety or stress' will only account for approximately 4 to 6 per cent of variability in an individual's actual level of stress. Therefore, there is up to a massive 96 per cent not accounted for by the personality test. A major factor here is that the very best of these types of tests are measuring an individual's likely personality traits but they do not measure their behaviour. For example, an individual who has high anxiety on a personality measure may not suffer from stress. Indeed, they may be highly driven to work long and hard, perhaps at some expense to their well-being but not necessarily.

The best professional use of these types of questionnaires is usually where they are used as a tool to elicit further information from a candidate regarding real world evidence of their behaviours. Alternatively, where they are used as a very small part of a decision-making process alongside other information such as personal statements or testimonials, etc. It is to be expected or hoped that the information from the UKCAT Non-Cognitive Analysis subtest will be used in one of these ways.

According to the UKCAT website the results from the Non-Cognitive Analysis subtest will be in the form of a band from 'A-E' as this reflects the nature of the questions. It is assumed that 'A' will represent a very high level of robustness, empathy and integrity through to 'E' representing a very low level of these attributes.

If you are interested to learn more you can access more information about personality testing by looking up 'personality tests' on www.en.wikipedia.org

Non-Cognitive Analysis subtest

The Non-Cognitive Analysis subtest is an onscreen test that will consist of a series of questions which will take no longer than 30 minutes to complete. The actual number of questions in not given on the UKCAT website but generally this type of 'personality' questionnaire would contain somewhere between 100 to 160 questions in the given timescale. This is only an estimate and the actual number of questions may be less. This subtest differs from the other four UKCAT subtests in that there are **no right or wrong answers.**

Response formats and example questions

Some questions will be based around a piece of text followed by statements which you will be asked to rate your level of agreement or disagreement with. Some questions will present statements of how you might behave or think in certain situations, and general statements about how you may feel about others. You will be asked to rate the truth or falsity of these statements according to your own beliefs and values. Some questions will present paired statements that represent opposing points of view and you will be asked to indicate your level of agreement on a scale between the two statements. The example questions on the UKCAT website www.ukcat.ac.uk will provide a useful taster of the format of the questions.

Example questions

The following examples are intended to provide a sample of the types of questions that will be asked. They will be followed by an explanation of which trait/characteristic they are attempting to assess (these will only be capsule descriptions). Most of the questions will be measuring a bi-polar scale, for example, 'low anxiety' as opposed to 'high anxiety'. It should be noted that both ends of each scale can have advantages and disadvantages given the demands of situations. As a 'lay person' in the field of personality assessment you may not always be able to link questions in this way and it is advised that you do not spend time pondering this when you sit the UKCAT.

Unlike the other four sub-tests it will be of no value to you to provide a set of scored practice items. However, the section following this one will provide you with useful tips on how to approach this type of questionnaire.

Example 1

I know I can do things better than most people.

False	Somewhat False	Somewhat True	True

This type of question is attempting to measure your level of self-esteem – a 'False' response would load onto low self-esteem and a 'True' response would load onto high self-esteem with moderators between.

People with high self-esteem are confident in themselves and their abilities whilst low scorers lack confidence and believe that they are prone to failure. Conversely, high scorers may appear to be over confident whilst low scorers may strive to do things better.

Example 2

I seem to have more bad luck than other people.

False	Somewhat False	Somewhat True	True

This type of question is attempting to measure your level of optimism – a 'False' response would load onto optimism and a 'True' response would load onto pessimism with moderators between.

Optimists are generally happy and cheerful and look to positive outcomes whilst pessimists can be gloomy or depressed and have a belief that fate dictates their future. Conversely, optimists may overlook some problems whilst pessimists may always be on the look out for what could go wrong.

Example 3

Are you easily annoyed if things don't go according to plan.

Strongly Agree	Agree	Disagree	Strongly Disagree

This type of question is attempting to measure your level of anxiety – a 'Strongly Agree' response would load onto high anxiety and a 'Strongly Disagree' response would load onto low anxiety with moderators between.

High scorers get frustrated when things go wrong and may worry or get stressed unnecessarily whilst low scorers are laid back and calm and do not have irrational fears. Conversely, high scorers may be extremely driven whilst low scorers may appear complacent.

Example 4

I would never lie or cheat even if the stakes were high.

Strongly Agree	Agree	Disagree	Strongly Disagree

This type of question is attempting to measure your level of what is often termed 'social desirability' or 'faking good or bad'. These types of scales are often used to indicate your level of honesty when completing the questionnaire – a 'Strongly Agree' response would load onto faking good and a 'Strongly Disagree' response would load onto faking bad with moderators between. This type of question often appears to be a trick question, which may lead one to believe that they should say that they never lie or cheat, but how realistic is this?

High 'faking good' may suggest that you have presented an unrealistic positive image of yourself whilst 'faking bad' may suggest that you have undesirable social habits. Conversely, someone with a high faking good score may really believe that they are more socially desirable than most even if this is unrealistic whilst someone faking bad may really believe that they should admit to human failings.

Example 5

The following item would require you to indicate your position on the scale between the two statements.

I hardly ever meet problems or tasks that I can't easily overcome or complete.

▦

▦

▦

▦

▦

I often meet problems or tasks that I find difficult to overcome or complete.

This type of question is attempting to measure your level of self-reliance or robustness – a response closer to the top statement would load onto robustness and a response towards the bottom statement would load onto a sensitivity/fragility with moderators between.

Robustness would suggest a capability to deal with almost any eventuality whilst sensitivity would suggest that some situations would be too overwhelming. Conversely, robustness may make someone appear to be to hard headed and task focussed whilst sensitivity may indicate a more tender-minded, intuitive approach.

If you are keen to complete a personality questionnaire and look at how the results are interpreted then there are several books and websites that allow you to do this.

Best approach when answering the Non-Cognitive Analysis subtest

■ answer the questions as honestly as possible, there may not always be sufficient information but answer the best you can

■ answer all the questions as they will all load onto the scales being measured (other than items that they may be trialling but you will not know which these are)

■ be spontaneous, your first response is usually a more accurate reflection of how you really feel

■ do not try to give the answers that you think are correct as this may produce a profile that is completely different to how you really see yourself

■ when answering questions that appear to be assessing integrity be realistic – these types of questions are often designed to load onto a scale that would suggest that you are attempting to present a more positive image of yourself than is realistic

■ do not spend time pondering items by trying to second guess what they might be measuring

■ do not try to answer from a particular scenario, for example, how you are with your close friends as compared to how you are at work, just give your most natural and spontaneous response

■ remember, you cannot cheat on this type of test; the result would be a profile that is not you and if higher levels of certain characteristics are deemed important in medicine and you do not possess them then maybe it would be an unsuitable career for you (this statement is of course subject to the comments made previously on reliability and validity and the use of the information)

Part III
Preparing for the BioMedical Admissions Test (BMAT)

The following chapters will help you to:

- understand the purpose and the format of the BioMedical Admissions Test (BMAT)
- understand the different sections and how to tackle them
- prepare for the test using BMAT-style questions.

The BioMedical Admissions Test (BMAT) was designed to help admissions officers cope with the problem of rising standards among medical school and veterinary school applicants. By examining the skills required to succeed in medicine and veterinary science, such as the application of scientific knowledge, decision-making and logical argument, they can differentiate better on paper between candidates who have the same top A1 grades.

The BMAT has always generated a lot of anxiety among students who are usually unsure of the standard and importance of the test. Now it has been joined in the admissions process by its new friend the UKCAT, its purpose may seem more unclear than before, especially as only a handful of UK medical and veterinary schools require it for entry to their courses (see Table 1). The first step to performing well in the BMAT is to understand its purpose and format. Then you can progress to familiarising yourself with the format of questions used and, finally, attempt practice questions and tests to build your confidence.

Whether you're reading this part of the book in a state of panic a week before the test or as a primer to familiarise yourself with the test, if you follow the advice given here you will not only alleviate a lot of your anxiety but will also pick up those extra crucial marks that can make all the difference to the success of your university application.

Table 1 Courses requiring BMAT

Institution	UCAS	Institution code
University of Cambridge	C05	A100, A101, D100
Imperial College London	I50	A100
Oxford University Medical School	O33	A100, B100
Royal Veterinary College	R84	D100, D101
University College London	U80	A100

Important note: if you are also applying to universities that require you to sit the UKCAT, you must sit this *in addition* to the BMAT exam.

Understanding the BMAT layout and scoring

The BMAT test has three parts and is two hours long in total:

Section 1	Aptitude and Skills	1 hour
Section 2	Scientific Knowledge and Applications	30 minutes
Section 3	Writing Task	30 minutes

These are all examined at the same time, but on separate answer sheets and with separate timings – hence you cannot run over on one part and make it up on another. Think of them as three separate exams taken during the same sitting.

Sections 1 and 2 are multiple choice or single best answer and will be marked by a computer. Some of you may not have met this style of answer sheet before, so it is important to familiarise yourself with it before the exam (visit the BMAT website at www.bmat.org.uk) so that you can appreciate the importance of recording the right answer in the right space. This may sound obvious but every year students miss out a question without leaving the correct space for it blank on their answer sheets. Only later do they realise what they have done, which inevitably leads to extra stress and mistakes.

Use an HB pencil for your answers (the propelling variety is good) and try not to rub out. If you do make a mistake, rub out your answer *completely* before you fill in your new answer. If you do not, the computer will read any remaining traces of your first answer and will assume you have chosen two solutions, thus invalidating that answer. This style of multiple-choice assessment is becoming increasingly popular among medical and veterinary schools, so it is as well to get used to the format now.

For Section 3 ('Writing Task'), use pen and write neatly. Watch your spelling and punctuation – there are marks for these and it would be silly to throw away marks on simple points like this.

How the BMAT is marked

For Section 1 ('Aptitude and Skills') and Section 2 ('Scientific Knowledge and Applications'), BMAT convert your marks into a score reported to the nearest decimal point on a nine-point BMAT scale.

For Section 3 ('Writing Task'), your paper will be marked from 0 to 15 and a copy sent to the institution(s) for whom you had to sit the BMAT in order to apply. Each essay is double marked and, if the mark is the same or a single point in difference, then the average is given. If there is a larger difference in marks, then it is marked for a third time. Obviously this is rather labour intensive for the BMAT examiners, but they do it to ensure that the marks are objective and that you won't be marked down just because one examiner doesn't agree with your arguments.

An important point to note here is that, unlike A-levels or GCSEs, you are very unlikely to score full marks on the BMAT. Figures 2, 3 and 4 show the scores from last year's BMAT students. As you can see, they follow a normal distribution, with very high scores being rare and low scores being even rarer. Section 2 scores (Figure 3) are much lower overall (probably due to the tight time constraint of this paper). Please remember that, however badly you think you will do on the test, it is almost impossible to 'fail' the BMAT – the test has been designed so that the average candidate for medicine, such as yourself, will score around 5.0.

Figure 2 BMAT Section 1 scores

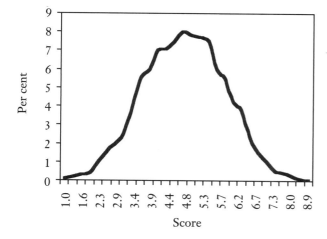
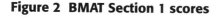

Figure 3 BMAT Section 2 scores

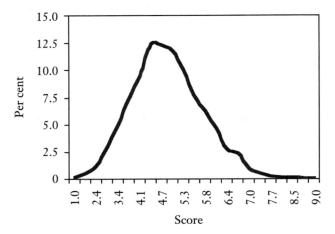

Figure 4 BMAT Section 3 scores

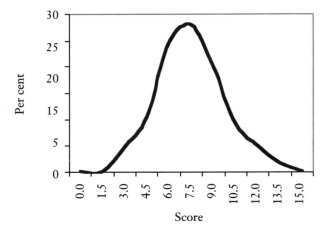

The BMAT examiners know that only a few very exceptional applicants will score higher than 7.0. There is, therefore, no need to panic if you find the exam difficult because it is more than likely that most other candidates will find it just as difficult. Some students do better on one section than on another, and it is for this reason that BMAT provide a breakdown of your scores so that your assessors can get a good idea of what your strengths and weaknesses are, rather than an overall average score that does not provide them with as much information. A downside of this, however, is that you cannot spend lots of time practising one part of the test in the hope that it will boost your mark; you need to prepare for all the sections of the test to the same standard.

For Section 3 (Figure 4) there is an even smaller spread of marks, with most essays scoring between 6.0 and 9.0. However, if you use the methods described in this book to practise for Section 3, you should score much higher than this (above 12.0). A small amount of preparation for Section 3 can really help to boost your mark here above that of the average candidate.

How your BMAT scores will be used

How your BMAT score will be used varies between universities. Some place a lot of weight on BMAT scores and use them as a criterion for inviting candidates for interview. Others use the BMAT as just one part of the application process, giving weight also to your personal statement, A1 scores and UCAS form when deciding whether or not to invite you to interview and offer you a place. So the BMAT is important, but don't prepare excessively for it at the expense of working on your A2s. If you get your UCAS form completed by the end of September, you will have a whole month to prepare for the BMAT.

If you are unclear as to how important your BMAT score will be for your application, check out the details in the prospectus or email the applications officer at your prospective university. If you do this before you sit the test you can, first, make sure you prepare appropriately and, secondly, you will save yourself a great deal of angst and worry if you think you have done badly on the day. The timescale for applying to sit the BMAT exam is detailed below. Check with your school or college if you are at all unsure about the arrangements.

BMAT application process: key dates for 2008

These dates are as listed by BMAT. Check their website regularly for any changes to the schedule.

19 September 2008
Closing date for requests for special versions of the BMAT paper (enlarged, Braille, etc.).

30 September 2008
Closing date for entries.

5 October 2008
Closing date for late entries (fees payable)

5 November 2008
BMAT test

30 November 2008
Results released to centres (and candidates).

11 January 2009
Closing dates for results inquiries.

The fee is £31 per candidate entered in the UK and £54 for international candidates. Late entry fee is £62 for UK candidates and £108 for international candidates. (This may seem a lot, but it's cheaper than the UKCAT.) You will need to be entered by your school or college and you must check that they can administer the test for you – let them know well before the end of September that you want to be entered for the test. Some schools and colleges have combined sittings, so you should check where you are meant to be sitting the test in advance of the day itself. If you have left school or college, you can make an application to sit the test at one of the open centres listed on the BMAT website.

In the following chapters the three sections of the BMAT test are examined in detail, with advice, worked answers and practice papers to test yourself. Don't try to work through the whole test in one sitting: work on each section of the test independently, in conjunction with the sample and past papers available on the BMAT website, until you are confident that you know how to tackle the type of questions you will meet in the real test. Familiarising yourself with the type and format of the questions and practising how to solve them are absolutely the best preparation you can do.

Chapter 13
Section 1: Aptitude and Skills

35 marks/60 minutes
Multiple choice or single best answer
No calculators allowed

During your time at university you will rely heavily on problem-solving skills, reasoning and analytical thinking in order to progress with your studies and to deal with the new ideas and concepts that you will meet. This is what Section 1 is for: it is attempting to find out if you have these necessary skills to cope with an undergraduate course in medicine, dentistry or veterinary science. So, although a lot of the questions may seem unrelated to what you have been studying in your A1 and A2 courses, the underlying skills needed to answer them correctly are very important.

You may be panicking because you think you don't have these necessary skills, or you may have heard that you can't practise for the test because you've either 'got it' or you haven't. BMAT itself says that 'An approach to developing these thinking skills can be taught, and the skills will improve with familiarity and practice. We encourage this because we think these skills are really worthwhile: they are useful skills in many walks of life, and very important for success in higher education.' So if you really want that university place and to do well once you get there, now is the time to invest some time in preparation.

BMAT goes on to say: 'What you cannot do is to be taught to answer as if you were a performing seal. There are no simple short cuts – you really do have to think the answers through.' While this is true to some extent, you can compare preparing for the BMAT with preparing for your GCSEs or A-levels. Normally, after you have finished studying the curriculum content, in order to pass the exam you work through practice and past papers. Doing the past papers won't teach you the knowledge or skills that you need to pass the exam, but familiarising yourself with the type of questions that are asked and figuring out how to apply your knowledge are a vital part of the preparation process.

This type of preparation is just what you should do for the BMAT. It is reassuring that the examiners themselves note there is no special 'trick' to answering questions: all the knowledge you require has been taught to you already at GCSE level. What you can do is get yourself up to speed by practising lots of BMAT-style questions so that, when you get into the exam, you can question-spot and recognise how questions should be solved.

Important note: on the BMAT website there is a list of recommended reading on how to improve your thinking skills. It is, of course, your own choice as to whether you read these, but I would advise you to steer well clear. These books are pretty wordy and not that useful for practising for the BMAT, especially if you have limited time on your hands.

Section 1 is worth 35 marks and tests:

- problem-solving (approx. 30 mins)
- understanding argument (approx. 15 mins)
- data analysis and inference (approx. 15 mins).

This means you have 60 minutes to get 35 marks (i.e. less than 2 minutes for each question). The marks tend to be split equally between the three question types, which are spread throughout the paper. However, the problem-solving questions take longer to read, so allow yourself a little extra time for these – but you will have to be speedy on the other types of questions.

There is no negative marking on the BMAT, so if you run short of time a guess is always better than no answer at all. For most of the multiple-choice questions you have at least a 20 per cent chance of getting it right. If you don't know an answer, fill in one answer as a guess and place a '?' by the side to come back to it later, if you have the time. Never leave an answer blank because you may run out of time at the end and thus never get the chance to make a guess at it.

However short of time you are, you must always read the question carefully. While the examiners do not set questions to catch you out deliberately, the questions often require you to perform a calculation and then give the remainder as the answer, or the questions may use different units from the answer choices. If you are rushing, you may not spot these nuances and all your calculations will go to waste. Also, beware of feeling relieved that the answer you have obtained is offered as a choice – the examiners also include the most commonly worked-out incorrect answers as possible solutions in the answer sets.

On the BMAT website you will find a number of practice papers you should do in exam conditions to get a feel for what's required of you. You can also visit www.ucl.ac.uk/lapt/bmat.htm. Here you will find hundreds of logic and problem-solving questions that test the same skills used in the BMAT – they even talk you through the solutions. Attempt the answer yourself first and then either pat yourself on the back or see where you went wrong. Rather than sit down and do them all in one mammoth session, do a few a day – that way you'll be consolidating your learning.

Below you will find worked examples of BMAT-style questions, with a step-by-step guide on how to approach them. After these you will find a BMAT-style test with answers and explanations of how to work them out. By working through these examples you should feel much more confident in your ability to tackle the BMAT.

Example: data analysis

1   The graph below shows how the flow rate of liquid out of a cylinder varies with time. The area marked B is twice as large as A. Which **two** of the following are false?

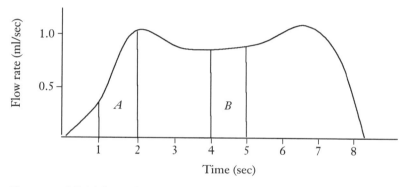

A   The rate of fluid flow after 4 seconds is twice what it is after 1 second.

B   The average rate of fluid flow is twice as great between 4 and 5 seconds, compared with 1 and 2 seconds.

C   The flow rate increases twice as rapidly between 4 and 5 seconds as it does between 3 and 4 seconds.

D   The amount of fluid flowing between 1 and 2 seconds is half as much as the amount flowing between 4 and 5 seconds.

How to solve it

First, work out what the graph is showing you – they even tell you: flow rate on the y axis, time on the x axis. Then, note that $B = 2 \times A$ (given) and realise that two of the possibilities are correct and that they want you to mark down the false answers. Don't be caught out! It is easiest to work out which ones are correct and then write down the other two.

A   The rate of fluid flow after 4 seconds is twice what it is after 1 second.
  We're dealing with rate of fluid flow, so read from the y axis. The flow rate at 4 seconds is around 0.9 ml/s; the flow rate after 1 second is around 0.3 ml/s. Because 0.9 is not (2×0.3), this is false.

B The average rate of fluid flow is twice as great between 4 and 5 seconds, compared with 1 and 2 seconds.

They have told you that the volume (area under the graph) of *B* is 2*A*. The three variables described by the graph are time, flow rate and volume. The volume has doubled, whereas the time period (1 second) is constant. Therefore the flow rate increase must be double.

C The flow rate increases twice as rapidly between 4 and 5 seconds as it does between 3 and 4 seconds.

The rate of flow is the graph line. It is flat between 3 and 4 seconds, and it's still flat between 4 and 5 seconds – i.e. the flow rate is remaining constant. Therefore this choice is false.

D The amount of fluid flowing between 1 and 2 seconds is half as much as the amount flowing between 4 and 5 seconds.

The *y* axis is rate of flow, the *x* is time. Remember that 'Rate of flow = Volume/Time'. Thus the area under the graph is volume. This is why they told you that *B* was twice *A*. So D is correct.

B and D are correct. Therefore you have to mark down A and C on your form.

The lesson here is that, although the questions in themselves are not difficult, there are lots of easy mistakes you could make in the heat of the moment, especially when you are under time pressure. Force yourself always to read the questions carefully before you jump in and solve them: you will save yourself a lot of time and will avoid making mistakes.

Example: problem-solving

2 Mr Jones has to renew the white lines on a 1 km stretch of road. Each edge of the road is marked with a solid line and there is a 'dashed' line in the centre. Drivers are warned of approaching bends by two curved arrows. Mr Jones will have to paint four curved arrows. The manufacturers have printed the following guidance on each 5 litre drum of paint:

Solid lines – 5 metres per litre.
Dashed lines – 20 metres per litre.
Curved arrows – 3 litres each.

How many drums of paint will Mr Jones require?

A 53
B 92
C 93
D 103
E 462

How to solve it

The solid lines require 200 litres for each side of the road (1,000/5).
The dashed line requires 50 litres (1,000/20).
The arrows require 12 litres (3 × 4).
Total paint required is 462 litres (200 + 200 + 50 + 12).

Beware! Most candidates at this point will go for choice E. The question asks how many **drums** of paint you require – you have worked out the litres required.

Total drums required is 92.4 (462/5).
You will have to round up to nearest drum. Therefore C is correct.

All the choices given here will seem correct – if you calculate the answer incorrectly! As you become more efficient at answering the questions, you will find time to double-check your answers. If a question at first seems too easy, look for the hidden twist. For example, forgetting to round up the drums may lead you incorrectly to select B, or only having a solid line on one side of the road will lead you incorrectly to select A.

Example: understanding argument

3 Vegetarian food can be healthier than a traditional diet. Research has shown that vegetarians are less likely to suffer from heart disease and obesity than meat eaters. Concern has been expressed that vegetarians do not get enough protein in their diet, but it has been demonstrated that, by selecting foods carefully, vegetarians are able amply to meet their needs in this respect.

Which of the following best expresses the main conclusion of the above argument?

A A vegetarian diet can be better for health than a traditional diet.
B Adequate protein is available from a vegetarian diet.
C A traditional diet is very high in protein.
D A balanced diet is more important for health than any particular food.
E Vegetarians are unlikely to suffer from heart disease and obesity.

How to solve it

These questions are tough, mainly because it takes quite some time to read the passage and the answers. The best way to approach this is to read the passage and then to pick holes in all the choices offered. Note that all the choices could be argued to be a conclusion – the question asks for the *best* choice (which is often the only one you can't pick a hole in). The conclusion is sometimes a statement in the text – although it needn't necessarily be at the end.

A A vegetarian diet can be better for health than a traditional diet.

This is the first line of the passage – think of news reports, which always have their conclusions at the start. Hold this one in reserve for now.

B Adequate protein is available from a vegetarian diet.

This is mentioned in the passage, but only by selecting foods carefully. It is doubtful if this is the main conclusion.

C A traditional diet is very high in protein.

It may well be, but this is an inference from the passage – vegetarians don't get enough protein so meat eaters must do(?) This is not the main conclusion here.

D A balanced diet is more important for health than any particular food.

It doesn't say so anywhere in the passage. Don't let what you know cloud your judgement about what the passage says. This is not the main conclusion.

E Vegetarians are unlikely to suffer from heart disease and obesity.

Be careful! Vegetarians are *less* likely, not *un*likely! There could be a 98 per cent chance, which is still less likely than 99 per cent, but still very high. Not the conclusion.

So, there is a choice between A and B. If in doubt, always go for the statement that has been mentioned explicitly in the passage. This may seem rather simple and make you second-guess, but remember there is nothing subtle about the BMAT! The best answer is A.

Now, try the practice test for Section 1. Check your answers after you have completed the entire test. There are fewer questions in this test than in the actual BMAT exam. This is so you can take your time with each question and focus on how you are working out the answers rather than using an element of guesswork. Make sure you are definitely happy with each question before moving on. Also included are explanations of how the correct answers were reached so that you can gain an understanding of how to tackle the questions and also learn from your mistakes.

Section 1 practice test

Time allowed: 1 hour

1 Mr Slicem-Dicem's private list decreased by 20 per cent in 2004, and by 50 per cent in 2005. By what % must he increase his private patient list in order to reach his original number of patients? Give your answer to the nearest whole number.

2 A dentist has appointments with 1,800 patients in a year. Twenty per cent of his patients are female, and 50 per cent of his male patients are over 60. He finds that, as a rule, one in 20 patients needs further dental work after they come for a routine check-up.

Assuming that all his patients attend for a routine check-up in a year, what is the number of male patients under the age of 60 who will need further dental work? Give your answer to the nearest whole number.

A 20

B 36

C 18

D 72

E 9

3 In the waiting room of the clinic, Tom places some toy-bricks in a pile. The red brick is above the blue brick, which is above the yellow brick. The green brick is below the blue brick and above the white brick.

The yellow brick must be:

A Below the white, but above the red.

B Above the blue, but not above the green.

C Below the blue, but not necessarily below the red.

D Below the blue, but not necessarily below the green.

4 A cable TV company charges a fixed rate for installation, and a rate for each kilometre of cable they have to lay to connect a house to the network centre. It costs the Abraham family £90 to install cable, and the Brown family £70. If the Abraham family live 10 km from the network centre, and the Brown family live 6 km, how much will it cost to connect my house, if I live 8 km from the cable centre?

Give your answer to the nearest £.

5 An elbow is a hinge joint and all hinge joints are synovial joints. The shoulder is not a hinge joint.

Which one of the following must be true?

A The shoulder is not a synovial joint.

B Every elbow is a synovial joint.

C Synovial joints are found only in elbows.

Questions 6 to 8 refer to the following information:

A medical student produced a report on the usage of local health facilities in the area. The bar chart below shows the reasons for people attending the Accident and Emergency department of a local hospital over a twelve-month period, with separate data for both men and women. The medical student was unable to collect any data regarding the number of men and women in the local population, so she is assuming that they are equal. Her consultant told her that the total annual A&E attendances are 5,000 per 10,000 men and 6,000 per 10,000 women.

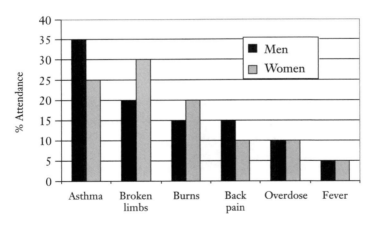

6 For both men and women, how many attendances are there per 10,000 for asthma?

A 3,000

B 1,500

C 6,000

D 1,750

E 3,250

7 Which problems did women have more than men in terms of actual A&E attendances? Mark all that apply.

A Asthma

B Broken limb

C Burns

D Back pain

E Overdose

F Fever

8 Which of the options in the table below contains the correct breakdown for A&E attendances for women per 10,000 per year?

	A	B	C	D	E
Asthma	3,250	3,500	2,500	1,750	1,500
Broken limb	2,500	2,000	3,000	1,000	1,800
Burns	1,950	1,500	2,000	750	1,200
Back pain	1,350	1,500	1,000	750	600
Overdose	1,100	1,000	1,000	500	600
Fever	550	500	500	250	300

9 If you drink too much alcohol and have a hangover, you may have a headache or tremors. Some, but not all, hung-over people with a headache also have tremors. Some, but not all, hung-over people with tremors also have a headache.

Which one of the options, A to F, correctly lists the following statements in order of their probability, listing the least likely first?

1 Someone suffering from a hangover will have a headache.
2 Someone suffering from a hangover will have a headache and tremors.
3 Someone suffering from a hangover will have a headache or tremors.

A 1, 2, 3

B 1, 3, 2

C 2, 1, 3

D 2, 3, 1

E 3, 1, 2

F 3, 2, 1

10 Two nurses, Amelia and Boris, each collect blood samples from my patients on the ward and do their rounds hourly. They are both as hard working as each other and blood samples are ready to be collected all the time. Unfortunately I can never remember at what times they visit the ward, so I just give the blood samples to the first nurse who comes along. Strangely, I discover over the year that Amelia collects more blood from me than Boris.

Amelia visits the ward at a minutes past the hour, and Boris visits the ward at b minutes past the hour. If Amelia visits the ward in the first half of the hour, which **one** of the following would explain the higher probability of Amelia coming to the ward first?

A $b > 30$

B $0 < (b - a) < 30$

C $0 < (b - a) < 60$

D $a > b$

E $a/b < 1$

11 The spread of HIV-AIDS is a subject which should greatly concern the human race. The march of this disease through our populations should be checked before it is too late. Our future as a species depends on the continued research and investigation into finding a cure, and we should not take comfort from the limited success of antiretroviral drugs. We should all give generously to charities which support research into this deadly disease in order to protect the future of our children.

Which of the following is closest to the underlying assumption in the passage above?

A HIV-AIDS is incurable.

B Antiretroviral drugs are ineffective.

C Donating to charity can help to cure HIV-AIDS.

D Charities provide most of the funding for HIV-AIDS research.

12 There are five houses on each side of a street, as shown in the figure below. No two houses next to each other on the same side of the street and no two houses directly across from each other on opposite sides of the street can be painted the same colour. If the houses labelled G are painted grey, how many of the seven remaining houses **cannot** be painted grey?

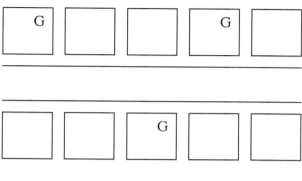

A one

B two

C three

D four

E five

F six

13 Tom and Joe shoot pellet guns at a target 2 metres away. Tom's gun shoots pellets which travel at 200 metres per second, while Joe's gun shoots pellets at a speed of 50 metres per second. What will be the time delay, in milliseconds, between the two pellets hitting their target?

A 40

B 20

C 10

D 3

E 30

Questions 14 to 17 refer to the following article:

Is bleach to blame for childhood asthma?

In a paper published this month, a group from Bristol University demonstrate a link between childhood exposure to domestic cleaning products and the development of persistent wheeze in children; a condition which often progresses to asthma. The study followed a cohort of more than 7,000 children until the age of 3.5 as part of the Avon Longitudinal Study of Parents and Children (ALSPAC). Analysis of questionnaires delivered both during and after pregnancy formed the basis of the study, with mothers being asked a number of questions regarding health and lifestyle choices. The participants were asked how often they used common household chemicals such as bleach, disinfectant, air-freshener and cleaning products, with their responses quantified to create a quotient of total chemical burden (TCB). The analysis suggested that no single product was solely implicated in the association with infant wheezing, and the authors were not able to determine whether the observed effect was due to in utero or postnatal exposure. However, given the strong correlation between prenatal and postnatal TCB scores found, and their association with persistent wheezing, it is likely that this represents postnatal exposure with a direct inflammatory insult to the airways (rather than a prenatal priming of airway inflammation in response to postnatal exposures such as airborne allergens). The headlines therefore centre on the statistically significant link between postnatal exposure to domestic chemical products and persistent wheezing illness in young children up to the age of 3.5 years, supporting an effect on the development of airway inflammation and asthma rather than a fundamental effect on airway development in utero.

With the incidence of asthma continuing to rise (the number of sufferers has tripled between 1970 and 2000), there has been much interest in the role environmental factors may play in causing asthma. Much speculation has centred on a possible link between household chemicals and asthma, especially given that the market for household cleaners has grown in line with the increased prevalence of the disease, and the observation that people,

especially mothers with young children, spend most of the day indoors. However, the Avon analysis is at odds with a similar study, published in 2003 which found no association between direct exposure to domestic volatile organic compounds and wheezing illness in children aged 9–11. In defence, the authors of the Avon study speculate that in this age category 'the majority of wheezing illness is likely to be established asthma and this may have a different aetiology to wheezing illnesses that develop in early childhood'. Another consideration is that, whereas previous observational studies have consistently identified a link between chemical exposure and asthma, few interventional studies have been able to document such an association. This may be due to participant numbers, duration of exposure or, most significantly, the observed association in observational studies could be confounded by a factor which is a determinant of asthma and is also associated with exposure to volatile organic compounds.

Such a confounding factor may be cleanliness itself. A popular explanation for the increasing incidence of autoimmune diseases in childhood cites the underexposure of children to environmental antigens whilst their immune systems are developing, so that they later develop diseases of atopy. Proponents of this theory cite observations that the increased incidence of asthma has followed the spread of urbanisation from the north southwards, and no doubt could interpret the results of the Avon study to confirm that a hyper-clean environment causes asthma. While these considerations could be integrated into the relationship between chemicals and childhood wheeze, critics point to countries such as Hong Kong, Sweden and Thailand, which have comparable levels of domestic cleaner usage and yet have the lowest rates of severe childhood wheeze. In a statement Professor Andrew Peacock, of the British Thoracic Society, said: 'More long-term studies are needed before we advise pregnant women to throw out all their air fresheners.'

Answer the following questions, assuming the information above is accurate:

14 Which of the following statements can we safely conclude to be accurate?

    A Being too clean causes asthma.

    B There are more asthma sufferers today than there were 30 years ago.

    C It is likely that just one product will be found to cause childhood wheezing.

    D Exposure to cleaning products in utero is more damaging than post-natal exposure.

15 The main message of the article is that:

    A Asthma is a dangerous disease in childhood.

    B There is a strong link between cleaning product use and the development of wheezing.

    C It is not possible to identify a cause-and-effect relationship between any factor and asthma.

    D Pregnant women should take care to avoid exposure to cleaning products.

16 If 10,000 people suffered from asthma in 1970, and the rate of increase mentioned in the article stays constant, how many sufferers will there be in 2030?

    A 30,000

    B 60,000

    C 90,000

    D 120,000

    E 150,000

17 Which of the following is not expressly mentioned by the article?

    A Hong Kong, Sweden and Thailand have the lowest rates of severe childhood wheeze.

    B There is much interest in the role environmental factors play in causing asthma.

    C The market for household cleaners has grown in line with the increased prevalence of asthma.

    D Children in the age group 9–11 suffer only from established asthma.

    E Previous observational studies have identified a link between chemical exposure and asthma.

18 Over the past 50 years there has been a rise in applications to read medicine at university. Because of this problem of increasing numbers, all students applying to read medicine in future should be required to sit a different exam from those that are currently used, in order to allow tutors to appraise students more effectively.

Which of the following are underlying assumptions of the above argument?

1 Exams performance can provide information on suitability for medical school.

2 The rise in applications is likely to continue.

3 Current examination systems are inadequate to assess suitability for medical school.

A 1, 2 and 3

B 2 and 3 only

C 1 and 3 only

D 1 and 2 only

E 1 only

19 £400 in a will is divided among five charities. The will states that no two charities are to get the same amount of money, and each is to have at least £20. The donations are to be given out according to the charity's size: the largest gets the most, the smallest the least. If these rules are adhered to, what is the largest donation that the third biggest charity can receive?

A 22

B 120

C 119

D 118

E 121

Questions 20 to 22 refer to the following information:

A medical school has student dormitories on both sides of its campus. The girls' dormitories are on the south side and the boys' dormitories are on the north side. Because of student protests, the Dean decides to integrate the dormitories and to move the first student on the alphabetical list, Miss A, from the south side to the north side.

The registry list of room, rent and test scores (before the move) is shown below:

South side (girls)			North side (boys)		
Student surname	Rent paid (£)	Test score	Student surname	Rent paid (£)	Test score
Adams	80	140	Hill	65	130
Brown	100	120	Ibrahim	70	145
Cowen	55	130	Jones	110	125
Docker	60	125	Kent	95	140
Evans	35	130	Long	75	120
Fetts	40	120	McNamara	70	125
Gower	50	145	Norman	85	130
Total	420	910		570	915

20 What is the average rent paid (to the nearest whole number) on the south side of the road after Miss Adams' move?

A 56

B 57

C 58

D 59

21 By how much will the average test score on the north side of the road rise after Miss A moves? Give your answer to the nearest whole number.

A 0

B 1

C 2

D 3

22 If all the rents rise by 5 per cent next year, what will the total rent bill be?

A £990

B £1,089

C £1,039.50

D £1,035.50

END OF TEST

Section 1 practice test: answers

Question number	Correct response	Comments	Marks
1	150%		1
2	B		1
3	D		1
4	£80		1
5	B		1
6	E		1
7	B, C, E and F	All correct for 1 mark	1
8	E		1
9	C		1
10	B		1
11	C		1
12	F		1
13	E		1
14	B	If plus any other answer, no mark	1
15	C		1
16	C		1
17	D		1
18	A		1
19	D		1
20	B		1
21	B		1
22	C		1

Section 1 practice test: explanation of answers

1 Mr Slicem-Dicem: 150%

His list originally was 100%. Thus in 2004 it was 80% (–20%) and in 2005 it was 40% (50% of 80%). In order to get from 40% back to 100% he must increase by 60%, which is a 150% increase on 2005 (60/40 = 1.5).

2 Dentist and his patients: B

1,800 patients, 20% female (thus 80% male); 50% male patients are over 60 (thus 50% of 80% of 1,800 patients are under 60); 1/20 consult; 1,440 × 0.5 × 1/20 = 36.2.

3 Tom and his bricks: D

The only way to do this one is by a diagram. Once you have done this, it is clear that the only possible answer is D.

Possible combinations:

R	R	R
B	B	B
Y	G	G
G	Y	W
W	W	Y

4 Cable TV: £80

Use an equation:

A $\quad x + 10y = 90$
B $\quad x + 6y = 70 \dots 4y = 20$

$\therefore y = 5$ and $x = 40$

My house is 40 + (8 × 5) = £80

5 Elbows and shoulders: B

Elbow = hinge = synovial
No other conclusions can be drawn.

A&E survey (6–8)

6 E

35% × 5,000 + 25% × 6,000
= 1,750 + 1,500
= 3,250

7 B, C, E and F

Multiply the percentages for men by 5,000 and the percentages for women by 6,000.

8 E

Looks a lot harder than it is. Work out the first illness value, then eliminate the others. Work out one more illness just to be sure you haven't made a mistake on your calculation.

9 Hangovers and headaches: C (2, 1, 3)

'Or' is more probable than specific illness, which in turn is more probable than 'and'. Watch that you list them in the correct order (i.e. and<specific<or).

10 Amelia and Boris: B

There is a lot of wording in this question, but many of the statements allow you to eliminate the given answer choices. Note that a and b are probabilities relating to Amelia and Boris.

A This choice does not explain why Amelia should come first as it is stated that blood samples become available at all times (i.e. not just in the first half of the hour).

B This choice is correct. Imagine Amelia comes at 29 minutes past (so within the first half of the hour, as stated). In order for B to be fulfilled, Boris must visit the ward between 30 and 58 minutes past (note the < symbol is used, not ≤) i.e. Amelia will always come first.

C Although this choice also describes the time condition as in B, it will not explain why Amelia comes first. If we use the example time for Amelia as in B (a = 29), the value of b could be anything between 30 and 88. Any value >60 would mean Boris visited the ward before Amelia, because the difference in minutes would mean he visits in the next hour, before Amelia.

D A lot of people will choose this one because it seems to describe that Amelia comes before Boris. However, the probability of Amelia and Boris visiting the ward is stated to be the same; what we are trying to find out is a description of why Amelia comes first (i.e. a condition of time).

E The same explanation as above holds for this answer; the probability of visiting the ward is actually $a = b$.

11 HIV-AIDS: C

The clue is in the last sentence when it says 'we should all give generously to charities… to protect the future of our children'. Thus it's therefore assuming that this money will help cure HIV-AIDS. The others aren't that convincing either. With this type of question, if you cannot decide between two answers, my advice is always to go with your original 'hunch': experience shows that it is generally correct.

12 Grey houses: F
The easiest way is to mark it out. Only one house is neither facing nor next to a grey house.

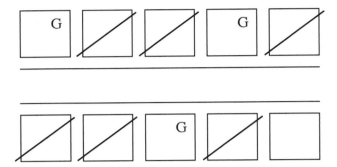

13 Tom and Joe: E
Speed = Distance/Time; ∴ $t = d/s$
Tom = 2/200, Joe = 2/50; 4/100 − 1/100 = 3/100 = 30 milliseconds

Bleach and asthma (14–17)
This is a long article, so look at the questions first; then you know what you are looking for when you read it.

14 B
B is the only factual statement from the paragraph, and thus we can assume it to be accurate (that's why the questions said 'assume the information above is accurate').

15 C
The article doesn't come to any conclusions regarding the link between cleaning products and asthma. Thus the other three statements are incorrect.

16 C
Easy: 10,000 × 3 × 3 = 90,000

17 D
Be careful: 'this age group is *likely* to suffer from established asthma'. This is not a fact expressly mentioned by the article.

18 Medicine applications: A
All of them are assumptions. Try to see if the article would make sense if you made each of the statements false.

19 Charity donations: D
Pay careful attention to the instructions here. Note it says 'the *largest* donation that the third biggest charity can receive'. This means you have to give 4 and 5 the minimum (£21 and £20, respectively). This then leaves you with £359: £121, £120 and £118. Note that it can't be £119 as then you would have to give two amounts of £120, which is forbidden.

Boys and girls (20–22)
This looks horrible, but most of the adding up has been done for you.

20 B
(420 − 80)/6 = 56.666 (57)

21 B
Before move: 915/7 = 130.7
After move: (915 + 140)/8 = 131.6
Difference = 0.9 (1)

22 C
Total rent = 420 + 570 = 990
5% = 49.50
Total = 1,039.50

Chapter 14
Section 2: Scientific Knowledge and Applications

27 marks/30 minutes
Multiple choice or single best answer
No calculators allowed

On first glance, Section 2 of the BMAT looks to be the most difficult, due to its reliance on testing factual scientific and mathematical knowledge. Remember that the standard is only GCSE level, and the examiners are looking for this level of ability in your tackling scientific problems rather than, for example, a detailed knowledge of the periodic table. Do not worry if you have not studied the subject further than GCSE level and feel a little rusty: as each of the subject areas is similarly weighted, you are likely to make up in one area what you lose in another and, with practice, you will be surprised as to how much of your past studies you remember.

A number of subject areas will not be tested (as stated by BMAT). These are green plants as organisms (i.e. no photosynthesis); products from organic sources; products from metal ores and rocks; products from air; changes to the earth and atmosphere; the earth and beyond; and seismic waves. Looking at what is left in the GCSE syllabuses, combined with what aptitudes the BMAT aims to test, enables us to make an educated guess as to those subject areas that will be tested in the exam, including the following:

- Human biology.
- Cells and cellular processes.
- Basic maths – equations, fractions, multiplication, algebra (remember, no calculators).
- Basic physics equations.
- Balancing chemical equations.

I expect these are all topics that you're studying or skills that you are using at the moment, but if you know you are weak in certain areas, such as your ability to do maths without a calculator or balancing equations, then get your old books out. Otherwise, what you really need to practise is time management – the challenge to obtain 27 marks in 30 minutes means you have to be speedy, accurate and decisive.

Again, note that there is no negative marking, so always give an answer. Work on 1 minute per question and, if you get stuck, move on after making a guess – you can return to it later if you have time. Remember that all the other candidates will be in the same boat as you time-wise, and an educated guess after reading a question will be better than going back through the paper in the last 30 seconds and filling in the questions you missed with wild guesses. There will also be lots of questions to which you know the answers immediately, and so this will give you a little more time for the questions you find more difficult.

I would advise against working out answers in your head as, under the pressure of the exam, mistakes are easily made and it also makes it difficult for you to check your answers if you have time on your hands later. The question paper can be used for all your working, but be aware that this is purely for your own benefit – you will only receive credit for answers correctly transferred and validly marked on the answer sheet.

Have a look at the past papers on the BMAT website to get an idea of what format the questions will take and what standard of knowledge you have to achieve. Below you will find some specimen questions to familiarise yourself with, together with their answers and solutions. These are just a flavour of the types of questions that could come up.

Some of the questions on the BMAT will be harder, some a little easier. Always look for the underlying rule or equation you have been taught that will allow you to solve the problem. Once you realise which equation or rule to apply, things will be a lot simpler. When you are familiar with the type of questions in Section 2, try the practice test at the end of this chapter and the ones on the BMAT website.

Example: maths

$$\frac{4x + 2}{2} - \frac{2x + 4}{7} = 9$$

1 x is equal to:

A 2

B 9

C 5

D 3

E 4

Answer

$(28x + 14 - 4x - 8)/14 = 9$
$24x + 6 = 126$
$24x = 120$
$\therefore x = 5$

2 Give the value of A in the figure below:

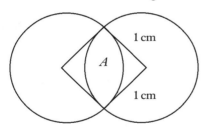

A $1 - \pi/4$

B $\pi - \frac{1}{2}$

C $1 - \pi/2$

D $\pi/2 - 1$

Answer

A bit tricky, but not if you realise that the area of a quarter of a circle is $\pi/4$ (πr^2 – always look at the answers to give you a clue). The area of the square is 1 ($1 \times 1 = 1$). Within the square there are effectively two quarter circles – total area $\pi/2$ ($2 \times \pi/4$) – which overlap giving the area A:

$$\pi/2 - A = 1$$
$$A = -1 + \pi/2$$
$$\therefore A = \pi/2 - 1$$

Beware answer C, which results from incorrectly rearranging the equation. As always, look for the trick to the question, and then solve it quickly and accurately.

Example: chemistry

$$\gamma CO_2 + \alpha H_2O \leftrightarrow \theta H_2CO_3 \leftrightarrow \delta H^+ + \beta HCO_3^-$$

3   Balance the above equation:

A $\gamma 3 \; \alpha 4 \; \theta 1 \; \delta 1 \; \beta 3$

B $\gamma 3 \; \alpha 3 \; \theta 3 \; \delta 3 \; \beta 3$

C $\gamma 2 \; \alpha 2 \; \theta 2 \; \delta 2 \; \beta 1$

D $\gamma 3 \; \alpha 2 \; \theta 2 \; \delta 2 \; \beta 3$

E $\gamma 3 \; \alpha 2 \; \theta 3 \; \delta 1 \; \beta 3$

Answer

At first look this seems very difficult – don't dive in and start trying to balance it! The equation is balanced as it is (no extra electrons), and so you just need to choose a solution that is a multiple of the original equation. B is the only one.

Example: physics

4   In the diagram below, what voltage must be applied for a current of 5 amps to flow through the bulb?

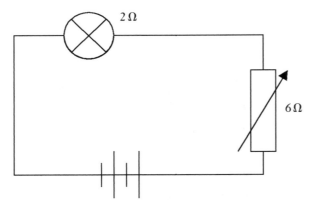

$2\,\Omega$

$6\,\Omega$

A   20 V

B   80 V

C   30 V

D   120 V

E   60 V

F   40 V

Answer

This is easy. It's a series circuit. Thus $V = IR$ (Ohm's Law) and you add the resistances:

$V = 5 \times (6 + 2)$
$V = 5 \times 8$
$\therefore V = 40 \text{ V}$

The only mistakes you can make is by multiplying the resistances, which would give you answer E, or by messing up your equation, which could give you variations of the other answers. The questions are only easy if you're careful and don't fall into the traps they leave for you when you're short of time and rushing.

Example: biology

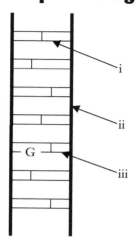

5 For the diagram above, select the correct labels for i, ii and iii from the list below:

A Nucleoside

B Adenosine

C Protein

D Guanine

E Polymer

F Sugar-phosphate backbone

G Nucleotide

H Cytosine

Answer

i G – nucleotide (beware nucleoside)

ii F – sugar-phosphate backbone

iii H – cytosine (C pairs with G)

Section 2 practice test

Time allowed: 30 minutes

1   Look at the figure of three intersecting lines below (the figure is not drawn to scale):

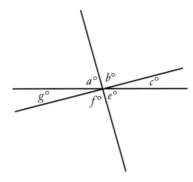

If $f = 85$ degrees and $c = 25$ degrees, what is the value of a?

A   60

B   65

C   70

D   75

E   85

2   In the figure below, triangles *ABC* and *CDE* are equilateral, and line segment *AE* has length 25. What is the sum of the perimeters of the two triangles?

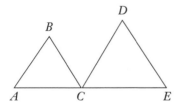

3   A solid block weighs 200 N and has the dimensions shown below:

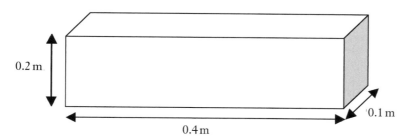

0.2 m

0.1 m

0.4 m

If the block can stand on any of its faces, what is the smallest pressure that the weight of the block will exert on the ground?

4   Below is a diagram depicting the knee-jerk reflex:

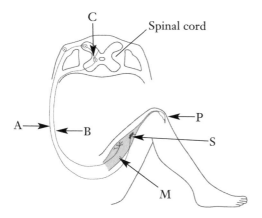

C

Spinal cord

A→

←B

←P

—S

M

Place the letters in the correct order to describe the direction of the nerve impulse:

A S, M, B, C, A

B S, A, C, B, P

C P, S, A, C, B

D P, S, B, C, A

E P, B, C, A, S

5   A resistor of resistance 1.0 kΩ has a voltage of 50 V applied across it. What is the current through it?

   A 0.05 A

   B 0.5 A

   C 0.005 A

   D 50 A

   E 5 A

6   The graph below shows the amount of water remaining in a tank each time a bucket was used to remove x litres of water. If 5 litres were in the tank originally, and $2\frac{1}{3}$ litres remained after the last bucket containing x litres was removed, what is the value of x?

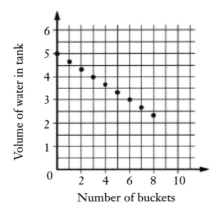

   A $\frac{2}{3}$

   B 1

   C $\frac{1}{3}$

   D $\frac{1}{2}$

   E 2

7 Which two of the following elements form compounds that are coloured?

A Copper

B Sodium

C Calcium

D Magnesium

E Iron

8 Circle the odd one out in the list below:

Amylase   Tryptase   Pepsin   Protease   Glucose

9 Balance the equation below:

_____ NaOH + _____ $H_2SO_4 \rightarrow$ _____ Na_2SO_4 + _____ H_2O

10 An ambulance is speeding towards the traffic lights and sees them changing to red. The ambulance is travelling at 100 m/sec. If it decelerates at a rate of 25 m/sec after the brake is applied, how long will it take to stop? Give your answer to the nearest second.

11 A consultant is boiling the kettle for his cup of coffee. The label on the kettle says it is rated at 2.5 KW. If it takes two minutes for the kettle to boil, how much energy is transferred by the kettle in the time it takes to boil?

A 3 KJ

B 5 KJ

C 30 KJ

D 48 KJ

E 300 KJ

F 30,000 KJ

12 Blood is pumped around the body by the heart. Select the correct pathway for blood after it exits from organ and tissues:

1 Pulmonary vein
2 Pulmonary artery
3 Right atrium
4 Right ventricle
5 Left atrium
6 Lung
7 Venous system
8 Vena cava

A 7–1–3–4–6–8–2–5

B 7–1–3–4–6–8–5–2

C 7–8–4–3–2–6–1–5

D 7–8–3–4–1–6–2–5

E 7–8–3–4–2–6–1–5

F 7–2–4–3–8–6–5–1

13 What is the total number of right angles formed by the edges of a cube?

A 36

B 24

C 20

D 16

E 12

14 The diagram below shows a pregnant uterus:

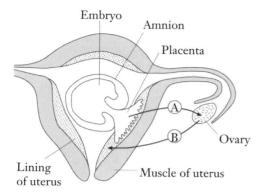

Circle the name of hormone A and draw a line under the name of hormone B:

Oestrogen   FSH   Adrenaline

Human chorionic gonadotrophin (HCG)

LH   Progesterone   Oestradiol

15 Iron sulphate and an odourless gas are produced by reacting which of the following together?

A Iron chloride + sulphuric acid

B Iron oxide + sulphuric acid

C Iron oxide + nitric acid

D Iron chloride + nitric acid

E Iron oxide + hydrochloric acid

16 The list below contains a series of statements describing the process of vomiting. Select which of the choices places these statements in the most appropriate order.

1   Contents of stomach expelled through mouth.

2   Signals received in vomiting centre.

3   Noxious stimulus from chemoreceptors and pressure receptors in central nervous system.

4   Reverse peristalsis.

A   1, 4, 2, 3

B   3, 4, 2, 1

C   2, 3, 1, 4

D   3, 2, 4, 1

E   1, 2, 4, 3

17 The graphs of the functions f and g are lines, as shown below. What is the value of $f(3) + g(3)$?

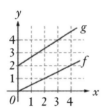

A   1.5

B   2

C   3

D   4

E   5.5

Section 2 practice test: answers

Question number	Correct response	Comments	Marks
1	C		1
2	75		1
3	2,500 Pa		1
4	C		1
5	A		1
6	C		1
7	A and E	Both correct for 1 mark	1
8	Glucose		1
9	2, 1, 1, 2	All correct for 1 mark	1
10	4 seconds		1
11	E		1
12	E		1
13	A		1
14	A = HCG; B = progesterone	Both correct for 1 mark	1
15	B		1
16	D		1
17	E		1

Section 2 practice test: explanation of answers

1 Angles along a line: C
   You know that angles on a line add up to 180 degrees. Angle e = 70 (180 – (85 + 25)). As $a = e$, angle a is 70 degrees.

2 Equilateral triangles: 75
   All sides are equal, so divide the 25 up how you like. If the triangle ABC has side of 10 and triangle CDE has side 15, then the perimeter is 25 + 10 + 10 + 15 + 15 = 75.

3 Solid block
   They would probably give you a choice of answers for this one, but it may be more fun to work it out yourself! The smallest pressure will result from the block resting on its largest area:
   0.4 × 0.2 = 0.08
   Pressure = Force/Area
   Pa = 200/0.08 = 2,500 Pa – always remember your units.

4 Knee jerk: C
   Patella tap (P) is sensed by the sensory nerves in the muscle (S) which is then relayed via the afferent nerves (A) to the spinal cord (C) and then down the efferent nerves (B) to the muscle (M), which contracts to move the leg.

5 Resistance and current: A
   Remember, $V = IR$
   50 = I × 1,000 (note the kΩ)
   ∴ current (I) = 50/1,000 = 0.05 A

6 Buckets of water: C
   A simple equation: $2\frac{1}{3} + 8x = 5$
   $8x = 2\frac{2}{3}$
   ∴ $x = \frac{1}{3}$

7 Coloured elements: A and E
   A knowledge one here. Think back to your practical sessions or, if stumped, then think sensibly – copper and iron are both coloured metals.

8 Odd one out: glucose
   All the rest are enzymes.

9 Balancing act: 2, 1, 1, 2

Take care with these sorts of equations. There weren't any charges to worry about, but there could easily be in a different question.

10 Speeding ambulance: 4 seconds

Acceleration/Deceleration = Change in speed/Time

25 = 100/Time

∴ Time = 4 seconds

11 Coffee time: E

Energy used (J) = Power × Time

E = 2,500 W × 120 seconds

∴ E = 30,000 J

= 300 KJ

Always think about your units for equations, otherwise you may end up a factor of 10 out.

12 Blood pumping: E

Before you look at the choices, work it out first, then see if your solution is offered. Otherwise, there's far too much potential for mistakes with numbers and letters, etc.

13 Cube problem: A

This is a spatial awareness test. There are the four right angles in each face of the cube, making 24 in total. Then there are also the right angles formed by the edges abutting each other, adding a further 12 to the total; 36 in all. See below:

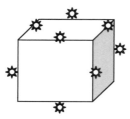

14 Pregnant uterus: A = HCG; B = progesterone
   HCG is secreted from the implanted blastocyst to inhibit further ovulation, while progesterone is secreted by the ovary to maintain the lining of the womb and to support the process of implantation. Unfortunately this is another knowledge-based question, although you could probably have a good guess from the answers supplied. If you have no idea of the answer, then the best thing is to guess and move on rapidly: spend the time on some of the questions that require you to work out the answer.

15 Chemical reaction: B
   Knowing it's a sulphate salt narrows it down, and the odourless gas can't be chlorine. A process of elimination.

16 Vomiting: D
   You may have to use your powers of deduction here if you have not studied this before. Try to work out what makes sense. Obviously, having the contents of the stomach expelled through the mouth is the final act, which narrows it to B and C. Then just decide that the signals are probably received before the action (reverse peristalsis) happens – solved!

17 Functions: E
   You can just look at the y values of the graphs at $x = 3$, but if you wanted to work it out then you can input 3 into the graph equations:

   $$g - y = \tfrac{2}{3}x + 2 = 4$$
   $$f - y = \tfrac{1}{2}x + 0 = 1.5$$

   Total of the two functions = 5.5

Chapter 15
Section 3: Writing Task

Choose one of three questions
30 minutes inclusive of planning and writing
Only one-page response allowed

Most BMAT candidates neglect to prepare for the final section of the test, either sacrificing the time for more preparation on the first two sections or believing that it isn't the type of task you can prepare for. If you have already looked at the questions in the specimen papers, you will have realised that they are very different from the type of factual essay you are used to writing in biology exams. Indeed, they seem more at home in a philosophy admissions exam than the BMAT.

However, the very fact that Section 3 is different from your normal A-level essays means that you should invest time in preparing for it – this section of the BMAT has been included specifically to test the skills that will be vital for your biomedical degree. An excellent answer on this section of the BMAT will demonstrate that you can:

- recognise and resolve conflict
- formulate and provide valid support for logical arguments
- consider alternative explanations for difficult ideas.

Looked at in this way, Section 3 suddenly seems a lot more relevant to your application than you probably thought it was. After you are happy with the question format and answer strategy of the first two sections of the BMAT, you should turn your attention to some proper preparation for the Writing Task. Time spent in preparation will reap bigger rewards than practising the same old multiple-choice questions again and again until you can do them in your sleep.

In order to prepare for the Writing Task, it is best to try to get your hands on the broadsheet newspapers and to keep up to date with the topical medical and ethico-legal debates. For example, there are always debates about whether the NHS should fund the purchase of unproven drug treatment regimens (think about the benefit for one versus the cost to many) or about court cases regarding ventilating terminally ill patients (which have to balance the right to life against the right to have a peaceful and private death). This isn't really the type of research that you can do on the night before the BMAT exam: not only will effective preparation allow you to incorporate convincing examples into your essays but it will also help you to think critically and to challenge information that is presented to you.

Over time I have seen that the best way you can prepare for this section of the BMAT is to invest in a notebook, divide each page in two and write down 'for' and 'against' arguments for each biological/medical/ethical/legal debate that you come across. Not only will this help you to clarify your ideas but it will also provide you with a fantastic revision prompt for the night before the BMAT. Although the issues you choose may not be asked about explicitly, you will build up a large library of examples, allowing you to answer the BMAT question that most appeals to you, as opposed to the only one that you could write two lines about.

As an added incentive, any time spent in researching for the BMAT won't be wasted. These sorts of ethical and biomedical debates make ideal interview topics, and interviewers will give credit to a candidate who can back up his or her arguments with elegant and relevant examples, compared with one who justifies his or her response with 'I just think it's wrong'.

However, in order to turn the brilliant examples you will collect into sparkling essays, you need to practise essay planning. Below you will find a breakdown of a BMAT-style Section 3 question that describes how you should order and arrange your essay and how to incorporate scientific examples effectively. I have also included in this chapter a Section 3 practice test, complete with suggested answers in the form of spider diagrams. You will appreciate that every answer is different, and it is how you incorporate your ideas into your essays that counts in the end (and in your score). If you work through these examples and practise arranging your answers as described, you can feel confident that you are effectively prepared for the final section. I cannot emphasise enough that you will receive a score directly proportional to the time and effort you invest in preparation, so make sure you prioritise wisely.

It is also worth having a look at the BMAT marking scheme for Section 3, available on the BMAT website. This will give you a good idea of what they are looking for, and of the differences between an answer that is average compared with an answer that is given top marks. Before you get stuck in, consider that the final section is as much a test of how well you can follow instructions as of what you can actually write. The following points may seem obvious, but the low average scores for the BMAT Section 3 suggest that perhaps they aren't.

Read the questions carefully

Take the time to read all the question choices and to decide which one you could answer the best. You would be surprised at the number of candidates who simply choose the first question on the paper (often in sheer relief that they can actually answer it). The question that seems impossible at first may offer a wealth of possibility on the second reading.

Plan your essay

You must *always* write an essay plan. Half an hour is plenty of time for you to write a single page of A4, so I would advise spending ten minutes of the time choosing your question carefully, and planning and thinking of examples. There is nothing worse than getting half-way through your answer and realising that you have completely run out of points to make, leading to you repeat yourself or leaving half of the answer space empty. More frequently, candidates run out of time or space on the sheet and have to miss out the conclusion, which is as vital a part of your answer as the examples that you give.

Planning an essay allows you to write an effective introduction and conclusion: there is no need to use the age-old trick of leaving a space at the start of your essay to write the introduction at the end if you have planned your entire answer in advance.

Answer the question

Always answer the question(s) asked. You have probably heard this a hundred times before but, unfortunately, too many candidates run off at a tangent and neglect to answer the question in hand (which scores them few or no marks). If they don't ask about it, they don't want to hear about it. That's not to say that you can't cleverly draw pre-prepared examples into your answer, but be aware that, unless you explicitly answer the question, and answer *all parts*, your answer will be marked little higher than an incomplete or absent answer. Try ticking the questions off as you answer them in your plan to ensure you incorporate all of them into your answer.

Avoid bias

Consider both sides of the question and/or argument. The examiners deliberately set questions that do not have a definite or right answer, which means that you have to present both sides of the argument. If you read some of the sample answers on the website you will notice that, often, they aren't very balanced and, as a result, they seem rather shallow and uninformed.

Include a couple of points in support of the argument and a couple against, and follow them up with your own opinions on the matter. Even if the question seems to ask just for your opinion, you must always present evidence as to why you think this in the form of examples, and always demonstrate that you have considered alternative answers to the problem. It is very important to show the examiner that you do not harbour any unfair prejudices – you do want them to let you into medical, dental or vet school after all!

Answer within the space provided

Use all the space provided but no more. Following instructions is important, and they have provided you with just one sheet of ruled A4 so that you write no more or no less. However, each year failure to plan the essay adequately causes many students to run out of space and to torture the examiner with teeny-tiny mouse-size script snaking its way up the margins, over the page and on to the desk. Unlike in A1 exams, the examiners aren't impressed by the expanse of your knowledge and will definitely mark you down for your failure to follow instructions and demonstration of poor planning. An excellent answer can be produced easily within the confines of one page, so when the lines stop, so do you.

First of all, let's consider how we would go about tackling some BMAT-type questions:

In the scientific world, advancements can only be made if mistakes are allowed to happen.

Explain what you think is meant by this statement: Can scientific advancements be made without mistakes being made first? What do you think determines whether a scientific outcome is a mistake or advancement?

Note that there are lots of 'mini-questions' in the main question, aimed at helping you to consider all aspects of your answer. The best way to cover these is to use them as the basis of your introduction, main body and conclusion. Also, make sure you take note of the trigger words in each question, which you may find helpful to underline:

Explain what <u>you</u> think is meant by this statement.

This is the perfect opportunity to grab the examiner's attention and acts as your introduction to your essay. Don't be afraid to state the obvious – they don't use trick questions. Below is one possible answer:

Scientific advancements arise as the result of many years of study and research and, in order to find the correct answer to a problem, you often have to make many mistakes first.

Although this is a good start, the answer fails to incorporate a personal touch (they are asking what you think after all) and also does not explain why mistakes *have* to be made (as opposed to the fact that they are just a part of research). A better answer would be something like:

I believe that this statement is describing the fact that, in science, there is no proof: a hypothesis can only be demonstrated to be wrong. In order to move forward, we have to demonstrate that all other theories are wrong. One way that this happens is through the process of making mistakes, and hence making mistakes becomes a vital part of scientific discovery.

This forms a concise and elegant introduction to your essay and will also lead nicely into some examples. It gives a flavour of what is to come and should tie in well with a conclusion. It also shows that you have planned your answer: it is often only when you start to plan examples for and against an argument that you realise what the original statement means.

Can scientific advancements be made without mistakes being made first?

This question should form the basis of the main body of your essay. It is just asking to be answered with lots of examples for and against (after you have done a few of this type of question, you will realise that they are all the same and the mini-questions will practically walk you through your answer).

It is probably easier to think of examples where mistakes had to be made for scientific advancement to be possible, and then to consider examples when they didn't. It may be that you find one half of the argument much harder than the other, and this will probably point you in the direction of what your conclusion should be.

This question is asking for scientific examples, but even if the question doesn't explicitly ask, try to choose examples that have some relevance to medicine or biomedical science – this is the BMAT after all! The best examples you could choose are the ones that could be argued both ways.

Scientific advancements with mistakes:

- *Drug testing*: at all stages of drug trials scientists are looking for side-effects and problems with the drugs. If there are, this means the drug is not fit for its designed purpose, which means there has been a 'mistake'. New drugs can only be developed by learning from these mistakes and refining the drug formula. Specific example: drug trial for Thalidomide led to the recognition that isomeric forms of drugs can be dangerous.

- *'Dolly' the sheep*: many failures and deaths of cloned animals occurred before the successful birth of Dolly, the world's first cloned sheep. Even then the scientists involved realised that she was born with the genetic 'age' of that of her cloned parent. This led to Dolly dying prematurely. However, these problems led to the scientists refining their cloning process and increasing their knowledge of cloning and what determines cellular ageing. Since then more animal clones have been created more efficiently and safely.

- *Transplants*: in the past, organ transplantation often led to rejection – the ultimate failure or 'mistake'. This prompted scientists to research why rejection was happening, leading to the scientific advancement of tissue matching donor organs with recipients.

Scientific advancements without mistakes:

- *Fleming's discovery of penicillin*: discovered penicillin growing in his laboratory; drug is still used today.
- *Early Renaissance scientists dissecting human cadavers pushed forward the knowledge of anatomy*: by actually observing the structures they could make no mistakes in describing them, although they did not understand all the functions of the organs or the changes that occurred at death.

What do you think determines whether a scientific outcome is a mistake or advancement?

This question is asking you to write a conclusion, incorporating the points you have already made. An average BMAT candidate will either neglect to answer this question properly or give an inarticulate answer. You should concentrate on two or three points you can use to draw everything together:

- Expected or not expected.
- Future work.
- Limits of current knowledge.

Here you have three examples of what determines whether a scientific outcome is a mistake or advancement. State them categorically and use your existing examples to back them up – this adds to the feeling that you have planned an integrated essay:

There are a number of factors that determine whether a scientific outcome is a mistake or advancement. First, it depends whether the outcome is expected or not expected. If, during an drug trial, it is expected that a reaction will occur, then if this reaction happens the outcome will add to scientific knowledge and become an advancement. If a reaction is not expected it could be classed as a mistake, but often investigation into why this mistake happened results in scientific advancement.

Secondly, it is often only future discoveries that confirm the status of a scientific outcome: there are always examples of fortuitous discoveries in science, such as Fleming discovering penicillin growing in his laboratory. However, it was only through future work, involving mistakes, that this discovery became a practical scientific advancement.

Lastly, the limits of current knowledge determine our perception of whether it is a mistake or advancement. It is only when the correct solution is reached that we realise where we had been going wrong, such as in the knowledge of organ rejection. It is only in retrospect and with the knowledge acquired from such experiments that we can classify them as mistakes. Therefore scientific progress relies on outcomes that are both mistakes and advances.

Notice how I summarised the questions in the last line of my answer. This is a trick you will all be familiar with from GCSE English, and it works here too in leading the examiner to believe you have answered the question more directly and concisely than you may have actually done. Just be careful that you don't rely on it solely as a conclusion: the examiners are familiar with this trick and will award you nothing for your efforts.

Have a look at the answer written by a previous BMAT student on the website. Try to count the number of points raised and the examples given. Often even the answers that receive the best marks only contain a few examples, so you can see how much they will do for your score. If you doubt that you could produce such a coherent argument, incorporating ready-prepared ideas will be much more effective than trying to think up examples on the spot. Also remember that exam conditions have the effect of making you write faster, so you don't need to worry about incorporating all your examples in the time allowed.

Now you have seen how to break down a question into its component parts, you should practise answering sample questions yourself, ensuring that all the questions are answered and that your essay hangs together well. After you have done a few questions you will realise that they all follow the same basic outline, with the multiple sub-questions acting as prompts for your introduction, main arguments and conclusion.

Once you are familiar with the approach to essay writing, rather than spending your preparation time in writing out page-long answers, I suggest you prepare spider diagrams to generate essay plans. This also has the benefit of being quick and easy to do in the BMAT exam itself, allowing you to draw links and contrasts between your arguments and to stay focused on the question. You can also tick off the points and examples as you progress through your essay, which helps significantly with time management.

Have a look at the example spider diagrams for the sample questions below to gain an understanding of how they can be used effectively. If you feel a bit unsure about essay writing, then you could use the example spider diagrams as a basis for your practice essays so that you can get a feel for how much of the contents you can incorporate into your essay in the 20–25 minutes of writing time you have during the exam. When you are confident in turning essay plans into great essays, then your remaining preparation can focus on generating spider diagrams and collecting examples.

At the end of this chapter I have included three more specimen tests for you to use either for spider diagram or essay practice, and you can also use the BMAT past papers as a basis for your spider diagrams. If you do use the BMAT past papers, remember that, while the style of the questions changes very little, the actual questions topics will change, so it isn't wise to spend too much time preparing answers and examples for the specific questions in the past papers.

Example essay questions

1 'Stop moaning! The pain is there to help you!'

What does the above statement imply? Give examples that illustrate how pain can be beneficial and others that illustrate the opposite. How can you explain the differences in the function of pain?

2 In the modern age of science, the laws of natural selection no longer apply to humans.

What do you understand by the statement above? Can you suggest examples where natural selection still applies and examples where it does not? What factors affect whether natural selection applies to a species?

3 Health and disease are points along a continuum, rather than separate states.

Explain what the meaning of this statement is. Do you agree with this statement? Advance arguments in support of and in opposition to this statement. What determines the balance between health and disease?

For   *Against*

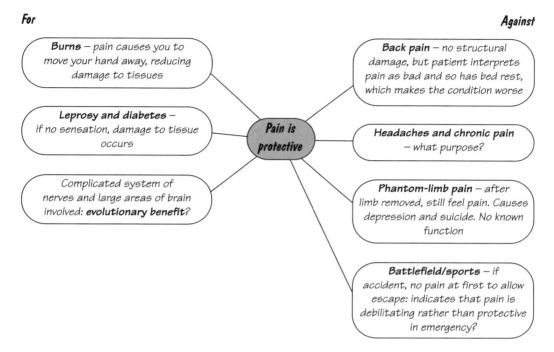

Example essay questions: suggested answers
1 'Stop moaning! The pain is there to help you!'

Statement implies

Pain is largely assumed by lay people to be a negative and harmful process, but the fact that complex pain pathways and mechanisms exist in humans may indicate it is protective and therefore of evolutionary benefit. The statement is also indicating that it is of a day-to-day benefit.

How can you explain the differences?

- Lack of knowledge (e.g. headache may serve some protective function).
- Pain may be so vital that mechanisms are 'hard-wired' into brain and independent of limbs, etc. (e.g. phantom limb pain).
- Psychological aspect of pain: different people in different circumstances feel the same pain differently (e.g. a broken leg on the sports field may hurt less than if someone attacks you).
- Different situations: pain sensation in the feet is wanted – lost in diabetes – but chronic pain that appears to serve no purpose is unwanted.

Yes   *No*

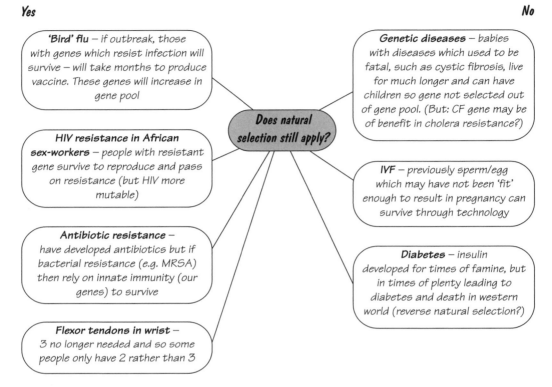

'Bird' flu – *if outbreak, those with genes which resist infection will survive – will take months to produce vaccine. These genes will increase in gene pool*

HIV resistance in African sex-workers – *people with resistant gene survive to reproduce and pass on resistance (but HIV more mutable)*

Antibiotic resistance – *have developed antibiotics but if bacterial resistance (e.g. MRSA) then rely on innate immunity (our genes) to survive*

Flexor tendons in wrist – *3 no longer needed and so some people only have 2 rather than 3*

Does natural selection still apply?

Genetic diseases – *babies with diseases which used to be fatal, such as cystic fibrosis, live for much longer and can have children so gene not selected out of gene pool. (But: CF gene may be of benefit in cholera resistance?)*

IVF – *previously sperm/egg which may have not been 'fit' enough to result in pregnancy can survive through technology*

Diabetes – *insulin developed for times of famine, but in times of plenty leading to diabetes and death in western world (reverse natural selection?)*

2 In the modern age of science, the laws of natural selection no longer apply to humans.

Statement means

Natural selection = Darwin's theory of 'survival of the fittest' – i.e. those best adapted to their environment survive and pass on their genes. In the modern age these rules may not apply due to medical and scientific support which effectively adapts the environment for us.

What factors affect whether natural selection applies?

■ Environment – the difference with humans is that we can change our environment to a large extent. But when the environment changes, it takes time for us to adapt.

■ Reproduction – now assisted (e.g. IVF: can increase disease genes).

■ Mixing of gene pool.

■ Mutation rate – much slower in humans – we have evolved mechanisms to prevent DNA mutation.

■ Time – generation time is much longer in humans; see changes slowly.

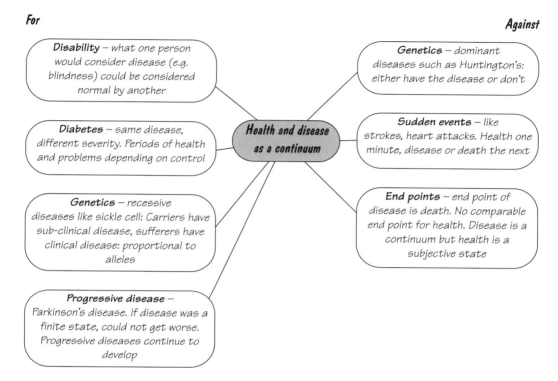

For

Against

Disability – what one person would consider disease (e.g. blindness) could be considered normal by another

Diabetes – same disease, different severity. Periods of health and problems depending on control

Genetics – recessive diseases like sickle cell: Carriers have sub-clinical disease, sufferers have clinical disease: proportional to alleles

Progressive disease – Parkinson's disease. If disease was a finite state, could not get worse. Progressive diseases continue to develop

Health and disease as a continuum

Genetics – dominant diseases such as Huntington's: either have the disease or don't

Sudden events – like strokes, heart attacks. Health one minute, disease or death the next

End points – end point of disease is death. No comparable end point for health. Disease is a continuum but health is a subjective state

3 Health and disease are points along a continuum, rather than separate states

Statement means

Health is often considered as the absence of disease. Hence one cannot exist without the other. It is the loss of full health that, for most people, constitutes disease, and the impact of this loss of health can vary greatly between individuals.

What determines the balance between health and disease?

- Individual perception.
- Perception of society.
- Medical advances 'normalise' some diseases so they seem less severe (e.g. diabetes).
- Nature and nurture.

Now you have some idea of how to break down the questions and understand how to use a spider diagram, have a go at creating spider diagrams and writing essays using the practice tests at the end of this chapter. There are no correct answers, but enlist your family, friends and teachers to help look over your essay plans and essays – after all, you want to try to achieve the broadest perspective on your outlook, and they will be able to suggest ideas and examples that you may never have thought of.

Although it is tempting to concentrate on the questions to which you already know you could give a good answer, attempt some of the ones that look less attractive. In the exam it will seem like all the questions are horrible and impossible to answer so, if you practise answering some that you find more difficult at this stage, you will be well prepared by the time you come to take the BMAT.

Section 3 practice test

Time allowed: 30 minutes

Practice test A

YOU MUST ANSWER ONLY <u>ONE</u> OF THE FOLLOWING QUESTIONS

1 'A cost to an individual can be justified by a benefit to the group.'

Do you agree with this hypothesis? Outline an argument in support of and in opposition to this statement. What factors influence the rights of an individual over that of the group?

2 You can only believe in what you know to be true.

What relevance does this statement have to scientific thought? Advance an argument against this idea. What other factors influence scientific belief?

3 The sequencing of the human genome is the most important scientific advance of the twentieth century.

Why is the study of the human genome so important? In what ways could the study of genetics be helpful in medicine and in what ways could it hinder advancements?

END OF TEST

Practice test B

YOU MUST ANSWER ONLY <u>ONE</u> OF THE FOLLOWING QUESTIONS

1 **The right to life carries with it the right to death.**

Discuss the implications of this statement. In what circumstances would you agree with this idea, and in what circumstances would you disagree? What factors would influence the possession of such rights?

2 **A patient's lifestyle choices (such as smoking, drinking alcohol) should not alter the medical treatment received.**

Do you agree with this ideal? Give examples of when medical treatment may be altered as a result of lifestyle choices. What factors determine whether treatment can be given?

3 **Medicine is an art form rather than a scientific discipline.**

Do you agree with this statement? In what ways could medicine be considered an art form, and in what ways could it be considered a scientific discipline?

END OF TEST

Practice test C

YOU MUST ANSWER ONLY <u>ONE</u> OF THE FOLLOWING QUESTIONS

1 **The ability to laugh is what makes us human.**

   What different meanings could this statement have? Advance arguments for the genetic versus the environmental effect on our personality development.

2 **All perceived benefits carry with them a known risk.**

   Discuss, with examples, whether this statement is true. How could we resolve the conflict between benefit and harm?

3 **Genes control our lives.**

   Explain what the statement above means. Advance an argument in support of and in opposition to the statement. How can we identify the role that genes play in our lives?

END OF TEST

Chapter 16
After the BMAT

Depending on the university you applied to and the style of interview, you may be asked about your essay when you go for interview, as BMAT sends each of the universities a copy of your Section 3 script along with your marks for Sections 1 and 2. The interviewers won't ask you about spelling and grammar, but they may ask you about your essay, especially if they thought it was well written or had some good ideas (which it should be, after all your hard work!). Therefore I would advise spending 10 minutes after you come out of the exam jotting down the spider diagram you used for your essay, along with the major examples. Not only will this keep your mind off which questions your friends got right and you didn't, but it will also serve as an aide-memoire when you are preparing for your interview, because it is almost guaranteed you won't remember anything about your BMAT test by the time your interview comes around a month or two later. It may well be that you never hear anything further about your BMAT exam, but 10 minutes spent now will at least stop you worrying about the possibility of having to talk about your essay later on.

Good luck for the big day. If you have prepared to the best of your ability, then you can be satisfied that you will fulfil your potential, however tough the exam. This effort and the skills that you learn will stand you in good stead for your future career.